THE
MAN PLAN

THE ULTIMATE GUIDE TO E. D. AND ROCK STAR ERECTIONS

DR. DAN LARKE

DISCLAIMER

This book is not intended as a substitute for the medical advice of physicians. The reader should regularly consult a physician in matters relating to his/her health, and particularly with respect to any symptoms that may require diagnosis or medical attention.

CONTENTS

CHAPTER 1

WELCOME TO THE MAN PLAN

Welcome! My name is Dr. Dan Larke, and I am thrilled that you have taken this first step to restore your sexual performance to a level that both you and your partner deserve. Do not make light of this significant first step, as many men will waste countless months and years in denial that anything needs to be done at all. So, while this is just the first paragraph, it is a significant milestone that you will look back on and remember the day you began to fight back against erectile dysfunction.

While my training in medicine has made me technically qualified to address this topic, it is my own personal experience and struggle that has allowed me to care for others with authentic empathy. I understand your pain, struggle, and embarrassment because I have lived it. What good would it do for me to tell you to be honest about your struggle if I am unwilling to do the same myself?

At the age of 39, it seemed as if there was nothing that life could throw at me with regard to my health that I could not conquer. In high school, I was an athlete who excelled at baseball, and I continued to play in various amateur leagues until my late 30's. Marathons and triathlons were part of my regular training regimen, and though I was pushing 40, I believed that I was in the best shape and overall health of my entire life. The Spring of 2001 would change all of that, and it seemingly happened overnight.

I started losing weight, which might sound like a good thing, but I went from a lean fighting weight of 195 to a weak 160 pounds in just four months. My symptoms of anemia, night sweats, and a general decline of health stumped many of the medical experts I consulted. Fortunately, we did finally find the root cause of my problem. Unfortunately, that root cause was stage 4 cancer, Hodgkin's Lymphoma. I had done everything to take care of my health to that date, and there was no logical reason that I could find as to why this happened to me.

Following standard medical protocol, I immediately had a chemotherapy port surgically implanted in my chest, and six months of chemotherapy seemed to pass in the blink of an eye. With great gratitude and a newfound appreciation for what it meant to be alive, I survived. The healthy version of the man that I had known my entire life did not. I felt like a man in his 70's, and I was emaciated, pasty grey, and a persistent brain fog hung over me that I thought would never end. Finally, and you may have guessed it by now, the penis wasn't working so great either, my friends.

The first step on the road to my recovery was an introduction to Naturopathic medicine. A friend in the medical field pointed me in that direction, and I'm beyond glad that she did. The results were miraculous. I started with a plant-based, whole-food diet full of fresh vegetables, fruits, and added some supplements. Within a few months, my mind had recovered, and the fog was gone. My road to physical recovery had begun.

You see, prior to my entrance into the medical field, I held a degree in aeronautical engineering and actually had the opportunity to design spy planes for a living. It turns out my background held great value in the medical profession because, as doctors, we are trained to understand the engineering of the human body. Our body is an amazing and complex machine. We've got hydraulics, pneumatics, pumps, electrical systems, wiring bundles, motors, levers, and a computer in our skull to top it all off.

When it came to erectile dysfunction, it was fascinating to explore what was happening to the machinery. Up to this point in life, my erections were just something that happened on autopilot and occurred without a hitch. So, what's happening to the body when it doesn't work that way? That was my journey that began this deep dive into erectile dysfunction, and that was the genesis of *The Man Plan*. A systematic and comprehensive approach to understanding erectile dysfunction informed by medicine, engineering, and personal experience to boot.

The goal of this book is to initiate a conversation between you and me. We'll talk openly, and we'll do it in a conversational manner that doesn't hinge too much on medical jargon. We will talk about the science behind erectile dysfunction, but most importantly, we will talk about a viable long-term solution in addition to the "quick fixes" currently being used. There are years and decades of sexual fulfillment ahead of you. You and your partner deserve a solution. I know that is true because I was in your shoes not too long ago. There is an answer, my friends, and you are one step closer to finding it.

Who is this book for? I'm going to assume that nearly everyone reading this book right now is in a few categories.

1. You are seeing the early signs of erectile dysfunction, and you've not quite gotten the nerve to see a doctor about it. I'm glad you're here, and you'll be happy that you didn't procrastinate too long before taking action.

2. You've tried treatments for erectile dysfunction before, but they didn't work, and you are desperate. I'm glad you're here too. I think you'll find that you may have been prescribed a magical pill too quickly, or that your doctor didn't entirely take the time to get to the root of the problem. Again, I've been here personally myself, and I won't leave you hanging. Figurative or literally, we'll get you back in action soon enough.

3. You are a committed partner to a man who struggles with erectile dysfunction and are seeking help along with them. Let me tell you that you are a keeper. Thank you so much for joining your partner on this journey. Armed with the information in this book, the two of you will be able to have some remarkably fruitful conversations together.

4. You neither struggle with erectile dysfunction nor have a partner who is struggling. You simply have some interest in the topic. Well, I'm glad you are here too, and you'll crush it on trivia night when erectile dysfunction comes up.

Regardless of why you are here, know how proud I am of you that you are taking this vital step. To get started, there may still be a few of you out there who wonder whether or not you really need to invest the time to read this book. So let's address that briefly and see if you need help with your erectile dysfunction. Spoiler alert, you do, and that's OK. Let's get started.

CHAPTER 2

HOW DO I KNOW IF I NEED HELP FOR ERECTILE DYSFUNCTION?

Well, for starters, you are into the second chapter of a book titled, *The Man Plan: The Ultimate Guide to E.D. and Rock Star Erections*. Don't get me wrong, this is a great book, but it is not exactly the type of book one reads for leisure. Something brought you this far, and if I had to wager, I would say that something is a struggle in this very area. You should be proud of yourself for coming this far, even if you can't quite yet admit that you need help. So let's drop the often dreaded term, erectile dysfunction, for just a minute and walk through a few scenarios instead. If one or more of the following statements applies to you, then you are in the right place, my friend.

My Wife or Partner Thinks I Don't Love Them Anymore

Unfortunately, the first casualty of a man's secret struggle with erectile dysfunction is his partner. That's not because she isn't getting what she used to get in the bedroom, but because she is left to think it is her fault in the absence of any additional information. This terrible side effect is often exacerbated by the timing of a man's struggle with E.D.. The romance and passion of a relationship forged in your 20's often gives way to the career and family obligations of your 40's and 50's. You'd like to say the bedroom is the only place where the shift in the relationship has manifested itself, but you and your wife know that this is not altogether true.

You used to be insatiable and frequently flirted with your wife for just the chance of an intimate connection. Sure, you'd like a romantic evening, but you've been known to share a quickie in the laundry room while the kids are eating lunch if you can pull it off. Now, you avoid touching her for fear that she will ask you for something that you can no longer guarantee. You stay up watching T.V. until you know she is asleep, or the pillow talk is minimized, and the sooner you roll over and go to sleep, the sooner your risk of embarrassment is over. She begins to think that she has lost you and wonders where it all went wrong. She is oblivious to the notion that it has nothing to do with her, and your marriage suffers as a result. If this sounds like your marriage, then this book is for you.

My Wife Thinks That I Am Having an Affair

The notion that you do not love your wife is bad enough; then again, a wife who thinks that you are having an affair can present an even worse scenario. The feeling that your romantic bond may be threatened by another person can be profound. Even though infidelity has not occurred, feelings of hurt and jealousy can trigger insecurity and dramatic conflict. The relationship can be irreparably damaged.

You used to be a sexual Tyrannosaurus, and now you seem to have no need? She's not buying that you are stressed and tired from your long hours at work. She starts to make up stories in her mind. If you are not getting it from her, then you must be getting it from someone else.

The irony is that you could be spending your evenings with your celebrity crush, but because of your E.D., you couldn't cheat if you wanted. Once again, your wife bears the burden for your secrecy, and you will, in turn, bear her burden if she thinks you are cheating. The terrible part about this scenario is that the paranoia could reverse, and you begin to fear that she'll want to have an affair. After all, if she thinks that you are cheating, would that not make her feel justified in doing the same? If your wife thinks you are cheating, or you think that she is cheating on you because of your E.D., this book is for you.

My Wife Thinks I Don't Find Her Attractive Anymore

The final dagger in your wife's heart is that you simply don't find her attractive anymore. She may be reasonably sure that you love her as you are a great husband and father. She may even believe that you would never cheat on her because you have always been a man of virtue. Thus, her only conclusion is that you simply do not find her attractive anymore. This is particularly devastating as she is well aware that she does not look the same as she did when you met. Having multiple kids has taken its toll on the body, and as much as she wants to present an attractive body image, she often looks in the mirror and weeps for what once was. The fact that you have no sexual interest in her only deepens the wound.

She doesn't know that she still rocks your world, but that you simply can't rock hers back. You've tried to be intimate, but your erections just fall short. Perhaps she even begins to reassure you that it's OK and that it happens to all men. You deny that's the problem, and thus, she is left to assume it is her. You've gone from having sex a couple of times a week to once a month, and now, even on date night is not a guarantee. This is not how you envisioned your marriage playing out, and it is breaking your wife's heart. If this sounds like a Friday night in your household, this book is for you. For that matter, this book is for your wife.

My Wife Says She is OK with Quick Orgasms, but I Know Better

Let's flip the script now and put the burden back on you. It may be that your wife is extremely secure and, in fact, so much so that she tries to comfort you with a lie. You see, erectile dysfunction is just one manifestation of this larger problem, and quick orgasms can wreak just as much havoc on a relationship. So when I say quick orgasm, I don't mean mastery of the art of the quickie that most married couples have obtained. Three kids running around the house and date night just got ruined because of a sick kid, but you still have to have it. So you and the wife stream a cartoon on Netflix and tell the kids you are going back to the bedroom to talk about what you are going to get them for Christmas.

Three to five minutes later, the task is done, and you can resume with your daily life. This is a good, and dare I say, acceptable quickie. However, on another occasion, two minutes into your anniversary get-away and you are already done is not the same thing. She loves you, so she tells you it's "fine." Yet, you know this is not true. You remember what it was like to go the distance and how she reacted when you did. Couples tell each other all sorts of face-saving lies, and this is no exception. She deserves better, and there was a day when you gave better. If this sounds like you, then this book is for you.

My Wife or Girlfriend Gave Me an Ultimatum to Get a Better Erection, or She is Leaving

Now this one hurts, fellas. Not only has your wife gotten better from you in the past, but she is now telling you that unless you get it up to par, she will get it from somewhere else. Ouch. Relationships can end for all sorts of reasons, but this is perhaps one of the more emasculating reasons for a man. If that is you, then don't fret. This is what this book is for, after all. However, many of you men may be on this road and don't even know it yet. She is getting frustrated, and though she may tell you that all is well, she is a woman, and she is a physical creature by nature. She might be too modest to say it just yet, but given enough time and frustration, this may be in your future.

It might seem shallow to many of those reading it, but there are countless books that counsel men on how to deal with relationships where women have a low desire for sex. Sex is a natural, enjoyable, and an important part of a relationship. Women are not wrong to want a fulfilling sex life. She is not being shallow to say that she is no longer getting what she had reason to assume she would receive in a relationship. Attempted sex is not sex. Cuddling is great, but it's not sex. Sexual acts of various natures may be enjoyable, but intercourse is still intercourse. This one hurts fellas, but if this sounds like you or you fear that this is in your future, then this book is most certainly for you.

I Never Knew I Had a Premature Ejaculation (P.E.) Problem Until My Breakup

Sadly, as much as men may try to conceal their problem with E.D. or premature ejaculation, your partner may also hide their problem with you. We talked about women saying they are OK with your premature ejaculation when we know that is not true. Many women do not want to seem shallow, so they mask an unfulfilling sexual life as a primary driver for a split. Meanwhile, the husband is under the impression that he has been some sort of sexual stud. That is until he hits the dating world for the first time in a long time. *"Ha-ha, that's it?"* Those are the last words a man wants to hear when he returns to the bedroom for the first time after a breakup.

Marriage is a beautiful thing, but routine and drudgery become commonplace as the decades roll by. For many married couples, sex becomes an obligation to get done rather than a joy to be expressed. When a husband suggests some intimacy and his partner responds with, "let's get it over with," and he responds with, "good enough," a recipe for monotony exists. You've forgotten that the rest of the dating world doesn't operate on that same scale of sexual currency. So if you are back on the market and are worried that your new female friends will have higher expectations than your wife of decades, then this book is for you.

I Can't Keep a Girlfriend because I Ejaculate So Quickly

You may remember your teenage years and the discovery that a quick orgasm seemed right around every corner. While this may seem entirely normal in our youth, it is not the norm for a man of advanced years to struggle with the same condition and certainly not with the same frequency. Not to mention that if you are hitting the dating scene with women in their 30's, 40's, and beyond, they have come to acquire certain expectations. I suppose you could still be a woman's first experience, in which case you can reply, "yes, honey, most men only last 60 seconds." However, I somehow doubt that is the case.

Whether you have never been married or perhaps recently divorced, premature ejaculation can be very damaging to the prospects of a long-term relationship. A woman is not confused by the knowledge that she is likely getting your very best during the courtship. So if your very best right now makes you a minuteman, then she is probably worried about a life of such performance. She is not being shallow, as sexual compatibility is a reasonable expectation of any long-term relationship. If you are worried that your quick-shot performance is hindering your prospects for a long and fulfilling relationship, then this book is for you.

Ever Since I Was Diagnosed with Diabetes, My Erections Have Been Poor

Diabetes is a common driver for erectile dysfunction, but the truth of the matter is that you can replace the word diabetes with most any inflammatory disease you want. As you will see in this book, there are a host of medical issues that can devastate sexual performance and take a significant toll on a marriage or relationship. I know you may believe that the condition is out of your control, and you are right to expect a certain amount of empathy and understanding from a committed partner. However, that doesn't change the facts on the ground. Or perhaps we should say, that doesn't change the facts between the sheets.

Lack of sexual activity and poor performance is an issue, whether it is spoken or not. You may be able to get an erection good enough to perform minimally, but a rock star performance seems like a distant memory. The bright side is that the penis is a human organ, and like most organs, it can be restored to a healthy state even after an illness takes its toll. You do need a plan, as simply popping a Viagra® or Cialis® may not always get you there. If illnesses like diabetes have wreaked havoc on your sexual life, then this book is for you.

I Have a Bend or Curve in My Penis

This condition (Peyronie's Disease) frequently comes up in conversations I have with patients about erectile dysfunction because men with such challenges are desperately looking for information and treatment options. The good news is that there are options for men experiencing a curved penis, and in many cases, they do not require surgery.

There is often worry or anxiety over sexual performance, along with a fear that a woman will be startled and find the misshapen penis difficult to accept. In addition, in many cases, there is pain and discomfort associated with the erection and a sense that the penis has lost length over time. We will be discussing the various treatment options for Peyronie's Disease at length, so if you experience E.D. challenges like this, then this book is for you.

Every Other Reason Under the Sun

We covered some of the top reasons that one might need this book. However, the truth is that there are a million more reasons under the sun why this book may be necessary to transform your sexual health. You and your wife may have a fantastic relationship, but perhaps you are just looking to give her a little more joy in the bedroom with an optimized erection. Maybe you are just curious about your own body, or you are the loving and committed wife/spouse/partner doing a little research for your man. If that's you, then congrats for supporting your partner in such a compassionate manner on such a difficult subject.

You are here for a reason, and we are glad that you are spending the time with us. Do you need help? Yes, the truth is that all men could use a little help in this area. As much as I've written about erectile dysfunction, I've found the information valuable in my own life when the stress or anxiety of the human experience starts to get to me. Whereas the human sexual clock has been extended by modern medicine, the clock is still not infinite. As a man, there is a sunset on our sexual activity, and as such, we deserve to optimize our performance to give and receive every amount of joy possible from this beautiful human experience. Is this book for you? If you plan to continue your sexual journey in life, then yes, this book is most certainly for you.

The Path Forward

In the upcoming chapters, we will be operating from the premise that there is hope for a healthy future for you and your sexual experiences. We'll talk bluntly, and we'll never pull our punches; instead, we will speak solutions over problems. We'll talk about the science behind it all and translate it into terms that you can comprehend. You are on the doorstep of a radically new you in the bedroom, and both yourself and your partner will thank you for your courage to move forward. Let's proceed, shall we?

CHAPTER 3

THE TRUTH ABOUT SEXUAL DYSFUNCTION

I am of the firm opinion that the first step on the road to recovering your peak sexual performance is understanding the biological and medical forces at play. This is not to make a doctor out of each and every one of you. Rather, I simply want you to understand that opinions or social stigmas about your inability to perform are irrelevant. One might have whatever opinion they want about gravity, but if you jump out of an airplane without a parachute, gravity will have its way with you, regardless of your opinions. So it is with erectile dysfunction. There are scientific forces at work that span both the psychological and biological worlds. Yes, it may be an awkward scientific topic because we are talking about your penis. Every penis joke you ever heard since your days in middle school comes to mind, but we are about to delve into the world of lab coats and science. I'll make it easy and fun for you to digest, but opinions are left at the door as the truth about erectile dysfunction will set you free.

What in the World is a Libido?

Libido could most easily be defined as sexual desire. A deeper dive would take a psychoanalytical approach and define it as the sexual drive's energy as a component of the life instinct. In Latin, the word means desire, longing, fancy, or lust, and we have the great Sigmund Freud to thank for popularizing its use in the modern lexicon. In layman's terms, libido is what causes you to cease one activity and engage in various behaviors that will hopefully lead you to sexual intercourse. In those terms, libido is a powerful force.

Libido will cause a man with little rhythm to consume multiple alcoholic beverages and gyrate on the dance floor like a human peacock. Libido will cause men to buy fancy clothes or a nice car with the hopes that he'll attract a partner who values status. Libido is one reason men who hate going to the gym will spend countless hours trying to look like a prime mating partner. Libido can cause men to fight other men in a show of force, and if the ancient writings of Homer are to be believed, libido even causes nations to war with one another. Many of the entanglements in which men find themselves are driven by libido because sexual desire is that powerful of a force. So, what happens when men would rather not do any of those things?

It is only when you realize what a primal and powerful force a man's libido is is that you become genuinely curious about why it fades. How is that a man who would previously climb mountains for the chance of sexual intercourse would now rather sit in his chair and not make the 40-foot trip back to the bedroom? "No thanks, honey, there's a History Channel special on the Civil War that I'd rather watch." It truly is a remarkable shift in the life of a man, and the cause can be either psychological or biological in its origin.

Psychological Stress - As I mentioned before, this is not an opinion. If you ever find yourself discussing your lack of libido with a friend or even your partner, they may offer a multitude of opinions, including that you seem stressed out. However, the biological impact of stress is more concrete. Our bodies react to prolonged stress in a variety of ways. There can be an immediate and sudden stressful event, such as a job loss. Then, there is chronic toxic stress such as financial insecurity, raising children, relationship challenges, or health concerns that take a toll over time. In either case, the body responds in kind.

It starts with the well-known "fight or flight" response that has been programmed in our DNA since the beginning of time. Functions like heart rate, blood pressure, and breathing become more intense, while non-essential functions, like sex drive, tend to be put on the backburner. I know you are thinking back to plenty of sessions of "makeup sex" that you remember as quite fantastic. However, stress causes your body to increase the release of hormones such as cortisol and epinephrine. Your body then taps the sex hormones to meet that demand, and voila, sitting in front of a T.V. trying to forget about your bills is suddenly more enticing than a romantic evening with your partner. Stress is just one psychological event with a biological effect. Depression, anxiety, and fear can all lead to a drastic reduction in sex drive.

Biological Responses - Another path to a drastic reduction in libido is the body's biological response to a variety of factors. Keep in mind that we are not yet talking about erectile dysfunction specifically. We are talking about a man's overall intent to pursue sex, regardless of his ability to produce an erection. Medications are a frequent cause of an overall reduction in sex drive as some medications result in a reduction of testosterone. You might know testosterone as the hormonal equivalent of "manliness." While that is somewhat true in a metaphorical sense, on a practical level, it changes the degree to which a man may desire sex.

Common culprits may include antidepressants, corticosteroids, opioid pain relievers, and chemo or radiation treatment for cancer. Again, the penis may work just fine in many of these cases, and an erection is entirely possible. You just have no desire to pursue that erection. When you are hungry, you will pursue food. When you are not hungry, other needs and desires seem more appealing. When you have a strong libido, you will do nearly anything to have sex. When you have a low libido, sex just doesn't seem that appealing.

The All-Powerful Erection

Once we get past the libido, the most obvious indicator that many men associate with a healthy sex life is the ability to produce and sustain an erection. This is a bit of a misnomer as one can engage in a powerful, intimate experience with a partner apart from an erection. However, if we are being honest, it is the struggle to generate and hold an erection that brought most of you here to *The Man Plan* in the first place. So let's talk about it candidly. The penis is a curious creature, and whether you realize it or not, you have been getting erections since you were a newborn. As a baby or toddler, it was more linked to your body trying out all if it's newfound functions. As a teenager, it was linked to a surge related to puberty, and that's why you would seem to get an erection at the most inopportune times. As a young man in your physical prime, you could seemingly conjure one up at will and recreate it almost as often as you liked. Now that I suspect some of you are a bit older, a powerful and firm erection is cause for celebration.

But yes, the inability to get or hold an erection is a tell-tell sign of erectile dysfunction. So let's briefly cover the biological details of an erection. You are well aware that the penis is the male sexual organ, but you may not be sure how it works behind the scenes. That it works at all is typically sufficient knowledge for men to operate. Inside your penis are two side-by-side cylinder-shaped chambers that run the length of your penis into your pelvic area. As a matter of fact, you only see about 40-50% of your total erection, with the rest buried within the body. They are called the corpora cavernosa, and they have a maze of blood vessels and specialized sponge-like tissue. Your urethra runs along the underside within the corpus spongiosum and is the tube that allows urine and semen to flow through. Two main arteries and a host of other veins move blood in and out of your penis. Nerves relay messages and tell your penis when to get ready for action.

That's why an erection starts in your brain, though at times, it seems like the penis is indeed the one in control of your mind. The science simply says otherwise. Your brain picks up something you see, hear, feel, or even smell and sends nerve impulses to your penis where it generates a chemical message in the blood vessels in your penis. Even a thought that recalls or imagines up any of these physical senses can create the same result. That's why when you find yourself daydreaming about your college days and spring break, you get a physical response in the present. Your arteries start to relax and allow the blood to flow into the penis. Pressure then traps it within the corpora cavernosa, and as your penis expands, you have yourself one healthy erection. When the brain signal stops, blood stops flowing in, or you reach orgasm, and the return veins open back up, you lose said erection.

Now a man can have varying degrees of an erection. If you have lived enough life, you know this by now. There were times where you could count on your erection to be solid and stable. Then, there are times where just enough growth to get it done was about all you could muster up. The truth is that many men who think they struggle with erectile dysfunction do not officially suffer from it. It is more likely a case of erectile dissatisfaction than dysfunction. Thankfully, we plan to cover it all with *The Man Plan*. There have been a variety of studies with conflicting results to measure the exact size of the average erection. Some men are looking for validation, while others are looking for hope. However, a 2013 survey posted in *The Journal of Sexual Medicine* put the average erection at 5.6 inches. Whether that encourages you or saddens you is entirely up to you.

In a later chapter, we will discuss Peyronie's disease in more detail. However, to advance the conversation, I'll cover it briefly now. Peyronie's disease refers to a problem caused by scar tissue or fibrous plaques that form inside the penis. The result is a curved erect penis as opposed to a straight one. It can range from a degree or two off-center to a sharp bend in one direction or another. It can result in sex that is painful for some men, and for others, it is the source of their erectile dysfunction. It might look different, but an erection by any other name is still an erection. It is also entirely possible to break your penis while it is erect. I know that is terrifying, but it is true. Not like a broken bone, but the blood vessels can rupture and cause some severely painful swelling. This most often happens during intercourse, where a "miss" is highly regrettable. Finally, I should also point out that you do not require an erection to reach an orgasm. It certainly makes it easier it seems, but science says a full erection is not required.

The Science of Ejaculation

For many men, the ejaculation is the culmination of the sexual experience. It marks the end of the sexual session, much to the dismay of many women hoping for a little more time and attention. Don't worry, fellas; we'll cover that as well. Let's start with a quick informational primer on your ejaculate (aka semen). What exactly is in this fascinating fluid, and where does it come from? Interestingly, your semen is comprised of fluid from four locations. During intercourse and as you become increasingly aroused, tubes known as the vas deferens will transport sperm (about 2-5% of your semen) from your testes to the back of your urethra. That sperm will be joined by fluid from the seminal vesicles (about 70% of your semen), then with fluid from the prostate (aka prostatic fluid, about 25% of your semen), and finally with fluid from the bulbourethral glands at the base of your penis (less than 1% of your semen) which helps to lubricate the head of the penis and clear the road for the mother lode. Together, they form what you inevitably see during ejaculation. The urethra can sense the buildup, and that's when the magic starts to happen.

At the height of your sexual excitement, your body sends signals through your spinal cord to tell the muscles at the base of your penis to contract in an immensely powerful and rapid manner. To be specific, this happens about every 0.8 seconds until the semen is forced out of your penis during the climax. Ejaculation consists of four distinct phases. Those are arousal, plateau, orgasm, and resolution/refraction.

Premature Ejaculation (P.E.) - When timed correctly, orgasm and the associated ejaculation can result in the culmination of a very beautiful experience. When it happens too early, as many of you know, you get the half-hearted reassurances from your partner that everything is "fine." Yet, you know everything is not fine, and that is why many of you are here. This is referred to as Premature Ejaculation, and it can be quite difficult for couples to face.

The inevitable question that arises is, "how quick is too quick?" The acceptable duration before ejaculation depends on the couple and is purely subjective. Simply put, there is no official rule on how long sex should last before ejaculation. Scientifically speaking, duration of sex is often associated with the IELT (intravaginal ejaculatory latency time), which is the time span from when the penis first enters the vagina and ends with the man ejaculating. It is worth noting that in 2005, a study was conducted of 500 couples from 5 different countries, and established that the median IELT was 5.4 minutes. That may help set you at ease when your friends brag about marathon sexual escapades, which is an outlier in the scheme of things. As many as 33% of men 18 years and older struggle with symptoms of P.E.

While the exact cause of P.E. is unknown, it is thought that a shortage of the neurotransmitter serotonin can play a role, as well as psychological issues such as stress, guilt, depression, and a history of sexual repression. Remedying PE can often prove quite elusive with options ranging from depression medications such as SSRI's to numbing creams for the penis, behavioral techniques, and professional sexual counseling.

Retrograde ejaculation is another way that male orgasm can go awry. This occurs when the semen enters your bladder instead of exiting through the penis. You can still reach an orgasm, but it is remarkably difficult to get your spouse pregnant when the semen heads to your bladder rather than her vagina. Signs that you are suffering from this condition are orgasms where you emit very little semen or none at all. People may refer to this as a dry orgasm or "shooting blanks." There are no other harmful effects apart from the inability to father a child or an emotional disappointment from you or your partner. Causes of retrograde ejaculation can range from the side effects of drugs used for an enlarged prostate, diabetes, bladder surgery, prostate surgery, and damage to the nervous system. Fortunately, the cause can usually be pinpointed with a thorough intake and physical exam, and in some cases, remedied.

Finally, there are those men who seem to be unable to ejaculate or take a significant amount of time to do so. This is often referred to as delayed ejaculation. It can be caused by a variety of physical conditions or medications and is generally not harmful apart from being a source of concern between you and your partner.

Delayed ejaculation can typically be broken down into several categories. Lifelong Delayed Ejaculation is present at the onset of sexual maturity. In contrast, Acquired Delayed Ejaculation occurs later in life for a variety of reasons. Generalized Delayed Ejaculation occurs regardless of sexual circumstances. Finally, Situational Delayed Ejaculation occurs due to the presence or lack of certain conditions. For example, some men can seemingly only ejaculate when they masturbate.

The Ultimate Orgasm

That headline may be a bit misleading, but it certainly caught your attention. The ultimate orgasm has been the quest of both men and women since sexual intercourse began. Achieving one on command has proved to be quite elusive, and there is no shortage of tips and tricks on how to get there. Some based on science and others based on aspects we'd rather not include in this book. However, an orgasm of any degree is not a guarantee in sexual activity, and for many men, an orgasm of any kind can be elusive.

The medical term for such a condition is Coughlan's syndrome. Specifically, it is the frequent inability of a man to reach an orgasm despite undergoing sufficient sexual stimulation. It is more commonly referred to as anorgasmia, and it can actually affect both men and women. Ladies, I'm sure there is some great literature out there for you on the matter, but this is *The Man Plan*. So let's jump right on behalf of men around the world suffering from this very condition.

Male anorgasmia can be quite a distressing event as it seems to mute much of the point of sexual intercourse. I should point out that anorgasmia is not the same as erectile dysfunction, though the conditions may co-exist. To understand anorgasmia, we have to dive a little deeper into the physiology of the male orgasm. As we mentioned above, orgasm is the third of phases that comprise ejaculation. It is important to note, as we discussed earlier, that not all men will ejaculate during an orgasm.

The orgasm is the byproduct of physical sensation or cognitive arousal, or some combination thereof. There are multiple nerve pathways, organs, and hormones involved in the process. Most men never think much of the science behind an orgasm, as the mere fact that they had one was sufficient to call the day a victory. Testosterone plays a central role by driving the libido while contractions of the muscles around the penis, anus, and perineum that propel the semen and give it the physical sensation. Meanwhile, the reward center of the brain is flooded with neurochemicals that enhance the response. When any part of this process is affected by physical or psychological factors, a man may find himself unable to achieve orgasm.

One can break anorgasmia down into one of two broad categories. There is Primary Anorgasmia, where a man can seemingly find himself unable to achieve an orgasm under any condition. Imagine being unable to reach an orgasm despite trying every effort under the sun. Next, you have what is known as Secondary or Situational Anorgasmia. This surfaces when a man can only reach orgasm under certain conditions such as masturbation or specific sexual acts. In either case, it can become quite stressful for a man as well as his partner.

Psychological Causes - It is often assumed that a man's inability to reach orgasm is due to some type of mental barrier. He can't get excited enough, or he can't focus properly to get it done. While those are generic assumptions often thrown out, there is some science behind why psychological factors would inhibit a man from reaching orgasm. Mental health conditions such as anxiety, stress, and depression may affect a man's ability to achieve an erection or reach an orgasm. Remember, erectile dysfunction and anorgasmia are two different things. Early sexual abuse or trauma can cause complications as well as negative or repressive attitudes about sex, where one feels guilty for having reached an orgasm. Anxiety over one's sexual performance can cause problems when trying to reach an orgasm, as the man is focused on the concern of his partner and is not enjoying the experience himself. So yes, the mind can play a pivotal role in the male orgasm, but there is some science to back up this claim.

Physiological Causes - Biology certainly plays its part in the male orgasm, and as such, it can be a primary driver as to why a man struggles to reach one. Most men have never heard of the bulbocavernosus reflex. However, if I told you that it is the reflex that triggers the anal sphincter to contract during ejaculation, then you would know exactly what I am talking about. Complications from prostate surgery or radiation to treat prostate cancer can affect a man's ability to reach an orgasm. More common conditions, such as uncontrolled high blood pressure or diabetes, can affect it as well. Prescription medications such as antidepressants (SSRI's) can affect men profoundly with anorgasmia, and the use of opiates, and even heroin, can play a significant role as well. Some doctors actually use SSRI's as a solution for premature ejaculation (P.E.). So it may seem logical that the use of these medications for someone without P.E. may be cause for difficulty in reaching orgasm.

The key to treatment is getting to the bottom of why any particular man is suffering from anorgasmia. This includes a thorough intake with attention to detail about psychological and physiological conditions, including the current use of any medications. The encouraging note is that once a cause is identified, there are a number of options one can pursue to treat the frustrating condition. So, it's not the end of the world for you or your partner. Sexual dysfunction comes in many forms, but the stress it puts on a relationship is nearly universal. Your partner may be understanding, but that emotional support does not change the physical realities at play. You and your partner deserve a solution, and The Man Plan will strive to guide you both towards the sexual satisfaction that may have been missing for some time. There is hope, and we are here to offer it to you.

CHAPTER 4

THE WOMAN/PARTNER RESPONSE TO ERECTILE DYSFUNCTION

As we enter this chapter, I want to throw out a quick disclaimer that may help advance the conversation. I fully realize that erectile dysfunction is a real problem that plagues relationships of all types. It is my goal that this book brings relief to couples participating in relationships that reflect the full beauty of the spectrum of sexual orientations and partnerships. Yet, to fully meet this need, we must address the biological and psychological reactions that are unique to the female gender. So, while we will be discussing the woman and spouse's response to erectile dysfunction in detail, please know that we are seeking to bring relief to all. Where you can apply the advice and direction universally, please do so. When we assume for conversation's sake that the spouse is a woman, it is merely to advance the dialogue with regards to the specific gender. With that said, let's jump right in.

A Season of Romantic Decline for All

Perhaps one of the most tragic elements deriving from erectile dysfunction is that it often occurs in a season of life where a decline in romance is usually deemed the norm. To be clear, one can be entirely romantic without sexual activity. So, I'm not talking about mere physical intimacy here, but romance and all the beauty that accompanies that. Physical activity is a contributor to romantic intimacy and not the sum of it all. You can remember meeting your partner, and perhaps you were even high school sweethearts. It was young love, and the world seemed to revolve around it. Now, your days are spent taking the kids from one activity to another and stressing over how to pay the bills. Hair is a little greyer, and things may jiggle now that were not meant to jiggle. Romance seems optional in this busy world, and as it goes for far too many, there just does not seem to be enough time or focus to pull it off. This masks and often extends a couple's recognition that there is a problem in the bedroom.

So, it is important to discuss and review a spouse's view on romance as the two are indeed linked. It is also helpful because a candid discussion on romance can help bridge the gap during the time that a problem with erectile dysfunction has been identified and a solution achieved. Many women will internalize a man's problem with erectile dysfunction and blame themselves. While some may withdraw, other women will try to enhance the romantic experience by doing their best to increase the erotic experience. If she thinks it is her fault, then she will try this new activity or wear that sexy outfit. She may see the performance issue as a reflection that she is not doing the right thing. Trying to bridge the gap in this manner is often less than helpful as erectile dysfunction has very little to do with not being turned on.

Another less than helpful approach is for the woman to tell the man that erectile dysfunction doesn't matter. She may see this as an act of love and compassion. However, we know that erectile dysfunction does matter in a relationship, and healthy sexual activity is a profound source of intimacy. So, it does matter, and saying otherwise only complicates the problem. However, it is vital for a man to recognize that both efforts are a woman's attempt to help. She simply does not have the biological experience to fully relate to the inability to get an erection. She has her own biological functions and experience, which operate differently. One not greater than the other, but that biological functions during sexual intercourse are separate and unique.

This is what makes open communication so important during a couple's struggle with erectile dysfunction. Finding a way to talk openly about the struggle allows each partner to have a certain amount of grace for one another. Exploring ways to pursue romance outside of the bedroom can help build intimacy and fulfillment while a solution is being pursued. However, this only works if the man has a clear picture of how his erectile dysfunction affects his partner. As mentioned earlier, erectile dysfunction most often occurs after the age of 40 and with increasing frequency as a man ages from there.

For many men, this may occur during the second or third decade of a long and loving marriage or relationship. Identifying the struggles that you are facing would be considered par for the course over a long relationship. Separately, identify what aspects are a direct cause of erectile dysfunction.

Finally, couples would do well to establish that saying "no" to sexual activity is not a judgmental or harsh response from either partner. A man who says no during a struggle with sexual activity has likely not lost all interest in his partner. A woman who says no during that same time is not entirely disinterested in her partner because he struggles to perform. Sexual intimacy can become a highly emotional and stressful experience during this season. Finding ways to pursue that intimacy outside of the bedroom is an important step forward. Seek to understand before you seek to be understood. There are countless ways to be romantic and sexual activity is just one of them. Unfortunately, this conversation often comes far too late, as we'll see in the next section. It requires a man to come to terms with his struggle, and denial is far too often the defense mechanism first chosen.

A Man in Denial is a Partner's Worst Enemy

Former Secretary of Defense and Marine General James Mattis once said of his Marines that there is no better friend or no worse enemy than a United States Marine. I'm here to tell you that a man's ego can very much be thought of in the same manner. Ego can drive men to accomplish unthinkable goals, and for many spouses, it was that swagger that perhaps attracted them to their man in the first place. Yet, when the body begins to decline in a manner largely uncontrollable to the man, the ego can quickly become a spouse's worst enemy. In this case, you could perhaps also consider the male penis itself as no better friend or no worse enemy. At one time, it was the participant of a fulfilling relationship. Now that it is struggling to perform, it is the source of great anxiety and stress.

Men are often conditioned from the onset of puberty to equate sexual prowess with masculinity. For much of their lives, sexual activity was as powerful a force as the need to eat or drink water. It is not an easy thing for a man to process when that changes, and unfortunately, he is often the last one in a relationship to come to terms with the fact that it is now a problem. A man in denial is indeed a spouse's worst enemy. He is unwilling to entertain the conversation, and though he can sense his underwhelming performance, his ego drives him to think that everything is just fine. The spouse knows that this is not altogether true. The spouse is faced with living with the reality of erectile dysfunction and all its consequences.

So let's start with the basics. While I don't have research data in-hand, I'm going to suggest that 99% of all spouses prefer a firm and powerful erection from their partner over a soft and flaccid penis during sexual activity. I'd go so far as to say 100%, but the realm of sexual preference always has its outliers. Men understand when their penis is firm and when it is soft. They are not confused by this matter, but ego forces them into a mental state that says this is just fine. In part, the woman or partner is responsible for this as they are not always quick to report an underwhelming performance. Faking satisfaction or an orgasm can often extend a man's delusional state while simultaneously building up the partner's frustration.

As signs of early sexual decline occur, men are also quick to dismiss the performance as one-off scenarios. Perhaps they had too much to drink that night, or they were simply stressed from work. Whatever excuse they may construct, the notion that they are about to enter a season of life where prolonged erectile dysfunction will be the new norm is not the first place they go. As they begin to come to terms that this is a more significant problem, many men are then quick to dismiss the potential decline as a sign of aging. Their first thoughts may turn to Viagra or similar medications that are not a long-term or definitive solution. The tragic consequence of this denial is often years or perhaps even a decade or more of sexual dissatisfaction within their partner. To say that this takes a toll on any relationship is an understatement.

Finally, we have to examine the mental and psychological toll that prolonged erectile dysfunction can cause in a partner. Many women who cannot biologically relate to the man's experience are left to make assumptions during this difficult season of life. They ponder that perhaps the problem rests with them. Maybe they are not quite as beautiful as they once were, or perhaps their partner has found his satisfaction elsewhere. Without the assistance of an open and candid conversation from their male partner, the woman simply cannot relate. Inevitably, this often leads the woman to withdraw from physical affection. If she is the cause of the sexual decline, she would prefer not to have to deal with the embarrassment.

There is great value and merit to a man who is courageous enough to start the conversation with his partner. A man who can recognize that this is a problem that may be out of his control has wisdom and intuition. A man beholden to memories of his former glory at his partner's expense demonstrates unprecedented selfishness. I do not mind putting that bluntly as I am convinced that those of you reading this text right now fall into the courageous category. I would encourage you to have grace for yourself if you have been in denial for a period of time. You are here now, and that is all that matters. Hopefully, you have not reached the point that we will discuss in the next section. If so, do not worry as you are still in the right place.

The Ultimatum to Perform or Get Out

We discussed how valuable it is for couples to talk openly and process their feelings and needs when they are affected by erectile dysfunction. We've also discussed how hard it is for many men to accept the fact that they are not performing as they once did in their prime. Sadly, for many men, even their best efforts lead them to the edge of the cliff. This is where a spouse has given a man the ultimatum to revive their ability to perform, or the relationship must come to an end. It is a tragic outcome and one that puts a man in quite a difficult spot, as he may not be able to meet the demand quickly enough, despite his best efforts. This is why communication throughout the struggle is so critical. However, it may very well have been such an ultimatum that has brought you to this reading. If so, let's discuss the partner's response and the emotions behind it.

Healthy sexual activity is an essential element of a relationship. Some couples may prefer more while others prefer less, but it is a critical component, nonetheless. Rather than respond with anger to a partner's ultimatum, it would be helpful to understand the emotions involved. On a basic level, there are the physical pleasures that are currently being denied to your partner. I would submit that this is not the primary driver behind the ultimatum. Many couples have meaningful and fulfilling sexual experiences without sexual intercourse. Moreover, a partner does have the ability to pursue pleasurable sexual experiences on their own. I would submit that the primary driver for a spouse's ultimatum to perform or get out comes from the lack of deep and meaningful intimacy that sex most often brings.

This is good news as this is something that you can pursue while you are seeking treatment or working through *The Man Plan*. However, it will require you to respond with empathy rather than anger when the ultimatum comes down. It can be quite hurtful, and the ultimatum itself can be a very traumatic experience. After the initial emotions calm down, and you have had time to process the experience, you would do well to attempt to put yourself in your partner's shoes. Is your partner wrong to desire and feel entitled to having deep and meaningful intimate experiences with the one they love? Was there a time in your life where you felt that your most primal needs were being denied, and did that cause you to make decisions you otherwise would not have made?

Part of accepting the fact that erectile dysfunction is a problem in a relationship is understanding just how powerful sexual desire can be. It presupposes that your partner has a need that you can no longer meet. They are not wrong to desire a solution, and they are not wrong to want a future with such deep physical intimacy. If you can reserve judgment for their response, which may seem extreme, it will allow you to focus more on the solution. This is also where separating normal relational stress from those stress caused by erectile dysfunction is helpful. Regaining the ability to maintain a firm and powerful erection will not solve those other matters, which may have led to the ultimatum. It is not a cure-all for a relationship, and both partners would do well to remember that. However, it can reduce a certain subset of stress that will allow the two of you to work through other issues.

In addition, this is also a time for you to examine your prior actions to address the problem. If you were still in denial, there is no denying that erectile dysfunction is causing problems when you are faced with an ultimatum. Looking back, can you honestly say that you worked diligently to address the problem? Were you fully aware of just how much this was affecting your partner? The ultimatum from your partner to restore your sexual performance or get out may indeed be harsh, but it can also serve as the wake-up call you have long needed. If this is what finally brought you to the point that you sought help, then you would do well to see this ultimatum for the blessing that it is. You, too, deserve a future with deep and meaningful sexual fulfillment. The ultimatum is the time to focus on the solution, and for most of you, that solution is within reach. It is not the time to simply give up on the relationship that you have long valued.

A Partner's Response is a Valid Response

In summary, this chapter was designed to help you understand your partner's response and hopefully serve as a catalyst for you to pursue the change that you both deserve. For women, understanding what you are going through takes a greater level of conversation and transparency. Yet, for all spouses, there exists the need for open communication. Both of you are right and just to desire deep romantic connections and physical intimacy that most partners enjoy. When that breaks down, it will have a lasting effect on the relationship. Regardless of how many times a partner tells you that everything is "fine," and it's not a big deal, it is a problem.

Thus, their response is valid. Even if the reaction manifests itself in an ultimatum to perform or get out, their desire for a better future is valid, and you would do well to receive it as such. Your solution will likely be different than another man's solution, but you can rejoice that a solution exists. Going forward, we will dig into the root causes and risk factors in more detail. We'll discuss the traditional approaches and why a more holistic solution is needed. Most importantly, we will discuss how to restore what your partner rightly and justly desires. You are less than halfway through the reading, and it is my hope that you are already feeling encouraged for the future. Your partner is not wrong to feel how they feel about it, and you are doing your partner to bring relief to their concerns. Let's carry on with the plan of the day and take the next step forward.

CHAPTER 5

RISK FACTORS AND CONTRIBUTING FACTORS OF ERECTILE DYSFUNCTION

Thus far in the book, we've briefly touched on the science of erectile dysfunction as well as the emotional aspects surrounding the man and his partner. Now it is time to dig into erectile dysfunction itself with a little more detail. Namely, what actually drives erectile dysfunction, and what are the risk factors? As you now know, there is not one singular cause. Consequently, there is not one unique solution. Later in the book, we'll talk about the need for a thorough intake to get to the bottom of your particular problem. Chances are, you've been to the doctor regarding this problem in the past, and if they didn't do a thorough intake, then they were merely guessing. You would have been just as well to throw a dart at the wall with some guesses on it. *The Man Plan* intends to be a little more precise. Our goal is to equip you with enough information that we encourage you to ask relevant questions and challenge your physician if you think something needs clarification. This is about your solution, and you are encouraged to be a part of that process.

Remarkably, erectile dysfunction has been a legitimate concern of men for thousands of years. Some of the earliest recordings were discovered in Egyptian tombs and on Greek vessel paintings. The record for the oldest reference resides in India, where an ancient Sanskrit text from around the 8th century B.C. put forward the root causes of impotence. I guess you could consider that text as the original "man plan." Roughly translated, it was suggested that the four fundamental causes of E.D. included 1) voluntary, 2) congenital, 3) early-onset, and 4) diseases of the genital organs. Thank goodness medical technology and science have evolved enough to narrow down the risk factors causing the problem. Not to mention that I imagine an 8th century B.C. version of an Indian penis pump would have been a brutal treatment option.

The fact that erectile dysfunction often occurs in older men has driven the prevailing thought that this is just a natural part of aging. We know now that this is not altogether true, as I have many patients in their 80s and 90s that have had wonderful sex lives with no issues. While that may not be an image you want to produce in your head, I applaud the men who pull that off. It is remarkable as we cannot emphasize enough just how fragile the symphony of events that lead to a successful erection can be.

This symphony includes everything from the emotional and mental arousal to the neurologic impulses coursing through your nervous system to the chemical reactions taking place at the speed of light in the blood vessels of your penis, which allow the vessels to enlarge and manifest the erection. I contend that there is always an underlying factor that plays a part in disrupting this symphony. So, let's run through some of these contributing factors that may be driving your erectile dysfunction.

Vascular Risk Factors

If you think about it on a surface level, it begins to make complete sense. The male penis is a tubular superhighway of vascular activity. So, it just seems logical that healthy vessels and proper blood flow are essential to a full and sustained erection. This is one of the most dangerous aspects of damage in our body as we age. Healthy vessels should be flexible and elastic, free of blockages, with a smooth inner lining to allow an easy flow of blood, nutrients, and oxygen to the penis and other vital organs. Atherosclerosis is perhaps the most common cause of vascular damage leading to erectile dysfunction. In layman's terms, this is when there is an obstruction of the blood flow to and within the penis due to a buildup of plaque in the vessels. Erectile dysfunction occurs when there is sufficient narrowing of the penile and cavernosal blood vessels to prevent a satisfactory erection. To put it bluntly, blood doesn't flow to your penis like it used to, and the vascular network in your penis is to blame. Think sexy thoughts all you want; if the blood doesn't get there in sufficient quantities, you are not getting the erection you want.

The most common underlying causes of atherosclerosis are factors such as smoking, high blood pressure, and high levels of glucose (diabetes), fat, and cholesterol in the blood. The alarming thing is that while most men seek help to resolve erectile dysfunction, they miss the big picture, which is that vascular disease is the most common precursor to coronary heart disease and heart attacks. This should also serve a wake-up call for men with E.D. to make changes in their lifestyle to prevent further damage. I'm going to submit that it is remarkably difficult to produce an erection once your heart has stopped.

What is it about these risk factors that actually cause atherosclerosis? The million-dollar word is "inflammation"! Inflammation is linked to almost every chronic illness, so let's cover it briefly. Inflammation is a normal part of the body's immune response to an illness or injury. When you have a wound or an infection, inflammation initiates your immune response to help fend off germs and facilitates the healing process. For short-term, acute conditions, such as traumatic injury, inflammation is helpful for healing. On the flip side, chronic conditions, with low levels of inflammation, it can cause damage to your blood vessels. This, in turn, promotes the growth of plaques (Atherosclerosis), which act to narrow the blood vessels, restricting the blood flow in the penis, and cause the vessels to stiffen and prevent vasodilation when you need an erection.

Smoking - In addition to causing a host of known illnesses such as lung cancer and COPD, smoking is indeed a contributor to E.D.. Specifically, nicotine and carbon monoxide are the primary culprits. When inhaled, they decrease the amount of oxygen that is carried in the red blood cells, cause inflammation, and increase vascular plaque, causing the arteries to harden, leading to high blood pressure, atherosclerosis, and ultimately poor blood flow to the penis. Nicotine also causes vasoconstriction, which also works against our need to increase the diameter of blood vessels to generate an erection. Recent studies showed that even in younger men, smoking produces signs of atherosclerosis in the arteries, which supplies blood to the penis.

Diabetes - As we stated above, Erectile dysfunction can also be a common complication of diabetes mellitus (aka hyperglycemia, high blood sugar, elevated blood glucose). Simply referred to as diabetes, this occurs when your body's ability to respond to insulin is impaired and allows too much glucose to remain in blood circulation. Ultimately this leads to inflammation in the blood vessels, which then leads to atherosclerosis. The end result being stiffened vessels and low nitric oxide, preventing sufficient blood flow in the penis for erections.

The connection between diabetes and erectile dysfunction has been known for quite some time. In fact, erectile dysfunction has been thought by some to be an early indicator of diabetes. However, at the end of the day, it all boils back down to the vascular system in your penis. Be it age, smoking, or diabetes; the vascular system is the primary culprit.

Cholesterol – While all cholesterol is not evil, too much of the wrong kind can add to the frustration of poor erections. It is essential for building new cells, insulating nerves, and even producing our hormones. While primarily made in the liver, we also take it in from food, such as milk, eggs, and meat. Too much of the wrong cholesterol may create a risk for vascular damage. In the presence of chronic inflammation, it can build up in the walls of your arteries, causing a reduction in nitric oxide, and you guessed it, atherosclerosis.

High blood pressure - Hypertension is a silent and insidious killer of your erection and your heart with the gradual increase of the pressure of blood flowing through your arteries. As a result, this high-pressure places added force on the artery walls. Over time, it can damage the cells of your arteries' inner lining. When the fats from your diet enter your bloodstream (we will get to diet later), they can collect in the damaged arteries and lead to atherosclerosis. That's right there it is again, that nasty 15-letter word, atherosclerosis.

The Venous Leak (Venogenic ED, or Penile Venous Insufficiency) - While the risk factors previously discussed are clearly vascular in nature, they are primarily associated with chronic disease and slowly affect the quality of erection over the years. Penile venous insufficiency is a form of vascular issue associated with reduced storage capacity, or the inability to store blood in the penis during an erection. Simply put, we need more blood flowing into the penis than flowing out. There is no consensus on the cause of this condition; however, in general, it is thought to be a defect in the connective tissue surrounding the penile veins. Men of all ages report this challenge, although it appears to be more prevalent in younger men who report symptoms early in age. The most common symptoms include a persistent soft erection inadequate for sexual intercourse, or position-dependent erectile rigidity (better standing vs. lying down). Challenges maintaining erections without constant manual stimulation, lack of spontaneous erections, and poor response to PD5E-inhibitors (Viagra and Cialis) are also examples of symptoms. Determining the presence of a venous leak requires a thorough intake, and testing may include an in-office test injection of medication to observe how the erection behaves over time. Treatment may involve the use of Trimix medication, an E.D. Ring, or, in some severe cases, vascular surgery.

These are certainly all common medical challenges with many men, although it is not all doom and gloom. The good news is that vascular problems are often treatable. You can't do anything to get younger, although these other contributors can be managed in a number of ways. While modern drugs may help to lessen the risks from these diseases, the ultimate goal would be to treat them with lifestyle changes, which we will address later. In the meantime, there is still hope and treatment for your erectile dysfunction. This is just one small example of why that thorough intake and proper evaluation is so important. Throw all the little blue pills in the world at a man with vascular problems to treat erectile dysfunction if you want. If you don't address the vascular issue, then you do not have a solution to the underlying cause.

Neurologic Contributors to Erectile Dysfunction (The Short Circuit)

As we learned in earlier chapters, the spinal cord, and nerves connecting your brain to your penis play a crucial role in an erection as well as ejaculation and orgasm. Thus, it makes complete sense that any damage to this system could cause problems with a man's ability to produce and maintain an erection. These neurological causes could stem from a variety of sources, including traumatic spinal cord injuries, nerve damage from pelvic operations, heavy metal poisoning, and even multiple sclerosis.

Essentially, the neurologic contributors interrupt the process of generating an erection by disrupting the communication from the brain to the penis, sort of like an electrical short-circuit in a machine. It would not matter if a man found himself in the midst of the most erotic scene possible if the brain cannot communicate that erotic feeling to the organ that matters. This is of particular importance as erectile dysfunction is thought by many to only affect men of advanced age. Yet, a man of any age can experience nerve damage or spinal trauma.

While neurological damage can be sustained during a surgical procedure to the spine, or from severe trauma, it is not limited to the back. Nerve damage caused by surgery and radiation to structures in the pelvic area, such as the prostate, can also facilitate neurological erectile dysfunction. Even though surgeons work meticulously to perform what we call a "nerve-sparing prostatectomy," there are still a relatively high number of men that become impotent as a result of nerves damaged during the surgery. It is possible that the erectile dysfunction from such a procedure may be temporary. As the man recovers from the procedure, his normal sexual functioning may return on its own as the nerves slowly regenerate. However, for many men, this is a long process wrought with much frustration and heartache. Because neurological causes can overlap with others, one should not assume that this erectile dysfunction is temporary and will restore on its own.

Hormonal Contributors to Erectile Dysfunction

Testosterone has long been thought of as the stuff of which manly men are made. This is part old wives' tale and part science, as testosterone does play a role in a man's sexual function. Yet, most would be surprised to find out that low testosterone is actually is only a minor contributor to erectile dysfunction, with more serious, underlying health issues as the actual culprit. Testosterone levels decrease naturally with age, as well as with chronic stress levels, so while low testosterone may not be directly linked to E.D., it does reduce our sex drive, energy level, and limit our ability to attain nighttime erections.

It is also worth noting that other hormone abnormalities can also contribute to low testosterone levels. Elevated prolactin (a pituitary hormone) and low thyroid (hypothyroidism) are two examples linked to low testosterone levels. It is also a little-known fact that Vitamin-D is actually a hormone. With this in mind, studies have shown there to be a link between low Vitamin D levels and low testosterone levels.

Many of you may have instantly run towards testosterone supplements to treat your erectile dysfunction only to be disappointed. That's why you are here today, and we will get you set on the right path. It is essential for men to have the sex hormone levels checked periodically starting in our 40's. This serves to establish a baseline and ensure that our hormone levels are optimized to head-off any potential issues with our sex life.

Medications as a Contributing Factor to Erectile Dysfunction

It is no secret that the side effects of many medications contribute to erectile dysfunction. While many drugs do include warnings on the label, there are many that make no mention of this. Here are some of the drugs that we know can cause E.D.: Blood pressure meds, Antidepressants, Antihistamines, Acid-reflux drugs, Anti-inflammatory drugs, Muscle relaxants, Opiate medications, Antifungal medications, Recreational drugs (alcohol, Amphetamines, Cocaine, Marijuana, Heroin, Nicotine)

It is important to note that we currently have an epidemic level of men with health conditions stemming from obesity that results in high blood pressure. So, it should come as no surprise that we see an equal epidemic of E.D. as a result of the untreated high blood pressure and the medications that actually treat it. Unfortunately, many patients are not informed of the E.D. side effects, and they only discover them after one repeated bedroom failure after the other. Now, imagine if you were not sexually active when you started HTN meds, and then some time down the road attempted sexual activity, only to discover E.D. You may not correlate the medication with the problem.

In that same light, we have more and more people diagnosed with depression and then provide antidepressant prescriptions that result in a less than favorable outcome in the bedroom. Military veterans with PTSD are given these meds to help combat stress and depression in their 20's and 30's and develop E.D. I have also had patients that don't understand why they suddenly develop E.D. during allergy season and never correlate their bedtime dose of antihistamines with lack of erections in the bedroom. Antacids (heartburn meds) are the 3rd highest selling over the counter (OTC) medications in the U.S., and we have a vast population of men with acid reflux purchasing these medications with a direct link to E.D. without knowing it.

Anti-anxiety medications can cause erectile dysfunction, as well. This is somewhat of a double-edged sword because anxiety can cause erectile dysfunction on its own accord. In this case, both the malady and the treatment are risk factors. Another common medicine-induced cause is conventional cancer treatments. That is often a life or death situation, so your sexual performance will take a back seat to survive. If you are about to undergo treatment for cancer, we encourage you to fight the good fight and live first and foremost. Just know that there his help for your erectile dysfunction on the other side of that battle. While it is well known that medications can cause E.D., it is often a sneaky culprit because the focus is usually only on the condition requiring medication. A full medication evaluation must be a part of any thorough intake process.

Lifestyle Contributors to Erectile Dysfunction

Beyond the medical factors at play, oftentimes, the simple lifestyle choices that we make play a role in erectile dysfunction. Those choices will have either a physiological or psychological affect. For example, if you want to improve vascular flow, it would be wise to quit smoking. If stress dominates your life, you may want to consider simplifying your routine and finding time to relax and decompress. Yet, at the end of the day, it all comes by full circle to the body and mind. Since we've already talked about smoking to some degree, let's jump to a few other lifestyle choices that can contribute to erectile dysfunction.

There are a variety of studies that have linked diet and erectile dysfunction. To be clear, this is not to say, "eat more of this and less of that." The science of dieting routinely changes as more evidence becomes available, and what was healthy today often becomes taboo tomorrow. So lest we lead you down the wrong path, we won't tackle it in that much detail. However, eating healthy foods (fresh veggies) has proven to reduce a variety of vascular problems caused by high cholesterol, high-fat content, high blood sugar, high triglyceride levels, and general obesity. Meaning, if you can't put down the hot wings and find a way to make exercise a routine part of your lifestyle, then you are putting yourself at risk for erectile dysfunction. Your partner may genuinely love the way that you look at any weight. Yet, if you can't reciprocate the love via healthy blood flow to your penis, then that is a problem. What you are eating at the kitchen table and the fast-food drive-thru can cause you problems in the bedroom. Pure and simple.

Stress and anxiety may not seem like lifestyle choices to many, but the choices we make in life can significantly reduce or contribute to a buildup of stress and anxiety. Yet, we all have stress, and even the calmest of us will report suffering some form of anxiety from time to time. So, what's the big deal? You have to remember that producing an erection results from a multitude of different body systems functioning properly. It could be physical stimulation, visual or mental stimulation, and even nocturnal stimulation during sleep. Each erection includes the nervous system, blood vessels, various chemical reactions, and hormones. Stress and anxiety have been proven to disrupt these functions in various forms. That crazy day at work, family stressors, financial issues, physical fatigue, and even the mental stress associated with having to perform sexually. We can also lose an erection in the middle of sexual activity if our mind shifts away from the task at hand and focuses on a stressor, even for a fleeting moment. The "Catch-22" syndrome can happen when you have an unsatisfactory incident in the bedroom, and then "it" gets in your head the next time you try to perform. It becomes a vicious circle of poor erections. Simply put, when we are stressed, the mind is preoccupied with these other events, which shifts our attention away from the sexual task of pleasing our partner.

So, when "today's" stress disrupts the nervous system, it can result in a weak erection tonight. But if your lifestyle includes daily stress that remains elevated for long periods of time, say years, you increase your risk of suffering from low testosterone, chronic inflammation, atherosclerosis, and, ultimately, severe erectile dysfunction. Lower your stress, and you lower your E.D. risk factor.

Finally, we will talk about depression. I was very hesitant to put depression under lifestyle choices as those who have suffered from deep depression can attest that it is no choice at all. However, seeking help and treatment can be a choice. Much like stress and anxiety, depression can lay waste to bodily systems necessary for an erection. It also proves to be a double-edged sword. It can cause a general lack of libido, and the absence or loss of a partner can serve to deepen the depression with feelings of hopelessness and persistent sadness. I very much wish that I could write something to lift you out of depression. You would do well to seek help for a thousand reasons unrelated to erectile dysfunction. Yet, if you long for the return of a fulfilling sexual experience, I can offer you hope. Seeking treatment for your depression can lift the effects it has on your sexual performance. Your depression may not be a choice, but you will need to choose to seek help if this is indeed the primary driver for your erectile dysfunction.

Nutrient Deficiency as a Contributing Factor to Erectile Dysfunction

Next, let's talk about nutrient deficiency as related to erectile dysfunction and sexual performance. While there may be some debate about nutrient deficiency as a direct cause of erectile dysfunction, there is no debate in the old saying that "we are what we eat." What we eat either provides our bodies with the critical nutrients, vitamins, minerals, amino acids, and hormones to keep the body operating optimally, or it doesn't. At the end of the day, a healthy and well-nourished body will always perform better than one that is not. We have already addressed the effects of diet on the risk factors of E.D., including diabetes and obesity. These lead to a multitude of health issues, including hypertension, high cholesterol, nerve damage, and ultimately vascular damage and our old friend, atherosclerosis.

A great deal of research indicates that Nitric oxide (NO) is one of the most essential molecules in the body. It is imperative for the proper regulation of blood pressure, prevention of cardiovascular disease, brain function, the immune system, reducing inflammation, and yes, erections. There have been over 60,000 studies done on nitric oxide in the last 20 years, and in 1998, The Nobel Prize for Medicine was given to three scientists that discovered the signaling role of nitric oxide. One of the most critical functions, as it relates to E.D., is opening the blood vessels to generate an erection. We have discussed that we need to get the blood vessels dilated in the penis to create an erection, and nitric oxide is the hero that makes that happen.

Unfortunately, as we age, a number of factors lead to the reduction of NO production and the reduced effectivity of NO in the body. These include obesity, chronic stress, lack of exercise, a diet low in nitrates and nitrites, medications such as antacids, and even the increased use of mouthwash. In short, obesity and stress lead to inflammation and vascular damage, which prevents the NO from doing its job to vasodilate. The poor diet, low in nitrates, prevents us from making sufficient nitric oxide, and the antacids and mouthwash prevent our body from processing the food rich in nitrates and nitrites to make the nitric oxide. The foods necessary to make the NO include dark green leafy veggies and beets. Another well-documented amino acid supplement that helps the body to produce nitric oxide is L-Arginine. This is a precursor to the formation of NO in the body.

As we discussed earlier, another nutrient deficiency that may be related E.D. is vitamin D. Often known as the "sunshine vitamin," research has shown a possible link between vitamin D deficiency and erectile dysfunction. We discussed earlier that vitamin D deficiency might be linked to low testosterone. A 2017 study published in the National Center for Biotechnology Information demonstrated that 35% of men with erectile dysfunction were deficient in vitamin D levels as well. Meanwhile, only 29% of men without erectile dysfunction reported the same. That may not seem like a wide gap, but it is significant enough to take note. This is important because vitamin D deficiency is easy to test for and remarkably easy to remedy. A modest change in diet, inexpensive supplementation, and sunshine can make all the difference in raising your levels enough to change your life.

Other vital nutrients to keep in mind are Vitamins B12, B3 (niacin), and Vitamin C. Sufficient levels of B12 help to keep the nerves healthy for proper erectile signaling. In contrast, excessive levels of B12 may actually be linked to mild E.D., so don't overdo those B12 energy shots, gentlemen. Low levels of B12 can be linked to excessive use of certain antacids (proton pump inhibitors), gastric bypass surgery, and even a vegan diet. Niacin (B3) has been shown to help improve E.D. in men with elevated cholesterol. Vitamin C supports the biochemical pathways leading to nitric oxide release and connective tissue production, which is essential in penile tissue health, increasing blood flow, and achieving erections.

If you have found your way to this book because you have erectile dysfunction, you will do well to address your nitric oxide, vitamin D,

Vitamin C, B12, and niacin levels with an appropriate supplement and diet modification. These are relatively inexpensive to check with a blood test. Even if they are not the singular cause of your erection challenges, they will certainly help your body function better in general.

Emotional Factors as Related to Erectile Dysfunction

The human sexual experience is one intended to be a pleasurable and beautiful experience. Unfortunately, this is not always the case for many men and women around the world. I would be negligent not to address the role emotional trauma can play in sexual activity and how events of the past can be a contributing factor to erectile dysfunction today. There is plenty of evidence today that links PTSD (post traumatic stress disorder) or other forms of psychological trauma to erectile dysfunction. This can be in the form of mental and physical abuse and also the horrid memories of military combat. This is beyond "basic" stress and even beyond prolonged periods of depression. This is deep trauma that manifests itself in the lack of one's sexual performance.

In a 2002 study in the Journal of Urology, nearly 85% of combat veterans seeking treatment for PTSD also reported symptoms of erectile dysfunction. That number is remarkable when considering that a mere 22% of the control group reported the same.

The result is that what should be a safe and healthy experience becomes a trigger for the trauma all over again. To the brain and the body, producing an erection is perhaps the least useful response at that time. However, recognizing that your trauma could be a contributor to your erectile dysfunction may be the final straw that encourages you to seek treatment. Much like depression, recovering from PTSD will likely take time, and seeking help from a skilled therapist is an important part of the healing. Your therapist will help to identify the triggers and reduce the severity of the symptoms of PTSD. There is no simple answer in the form of a pill or treatment protocol to resolve the PTSD and, ultimately, the erectile dysfunction. You did not deserve the trauma you experienced, but you do deserve a fulfilling and meaningful future where healthy sexual activity is a fulfilling part of your life.

In Summary

There exists a wide variety of risk factors and contributors to erectile dysfunction. This is why it pains me that far too often; the solution is an Rx for a quick blue pill that is treated as a cure-all solution. The body and the mind simply do not work that way. Moreover, treating erectile dysfunction with a quick prescription may mask the fact that your body is trying to alert you to a more significant problem. You need a thorough intake that results in a comprehensive solution to your erectile dysfunction. Anything less simply will not do. *The Man Plan* leaves nothing to chance. So now that we've covered some common risk factors let's discuss some of the common approaches to treatment.

CHAPTER 6

CONVENTIONAL APPROACHES TO TREATING ERECTILE DYSFUNCTION

If treating erectile dysfunction were so easy, there would not be much of an industry for doing so, and this entire book would be null and void. Yet, far too many men and women believe there is a magic pill that will solve all of their problems. This is partly due to the popularization of "the little blue pill" and part due to the fact that people long for simple solutions. They want it to be true whether the science supports them or not. This is somewhat tragic because, by the time a man musters enough courage to reach out for medical help for their erectile dysfunction, they deserve a better response. So, we'll cover some of the most conventional approaches for treating erectile dysfunction. The purpose is not to discount these methods as there are men who do indeed find relief from these treatments. Instead, the goal is to equip you with what you need to decide whether your doctors have fully considered the scope of your problem. Or are they are merely trying to send you off with a quick solution to a very uncomfortable topic. One of these approaches may be right for you, but to assume that is the best fit right out of the gates can be dangerous and negligent in my professional opinion.

The Magic Pill (aka PDE5-Inhibitors)

It is an all too familiar story, but it may very have been the narrative that drove you to this reading. You've known about your erectile dysfunction for a while, though denial has forced you to do nothing about it. Perhaps it was an ultimatum from your partner or just one too many date nights ruined, but kudos to you for finally reaching out to a medical professional for help. In most cases, this is your family doctor or general practitioner (GP). In some instances, you may seek the input from a Urologist or even call one of those E.D. clinics that advertise on the radio or has a late-night infomercial. Your reward for such courage is generally a generalist that does not take sufficient time to fully evaluate your situation, may not be fully informed on all the nuances of E.D., or in many cases, is simply uncomfortable discussing the topic.

With this in mind, they reach for their trusty prescription pad to write an Rx for Viagra (Sildenafil), Cialis (Tadalafil). These drugs are classified as PDE5 inhibitors (phosphodiesterase type 5 inhibitors). In a nutshell, these drugs assist the blood vessels in your penis in remaining dilated longer during sex. Now, the truth of the matter is that this is a none too pleasant conversation for you as well. At the first mention of a "magic pill," you say yes, grab the prescription, and then run for the door. The doctor may not fully cover the possible side effects, and you are not in a state of mind to want to hear them. No one can blame you, but the doctor who swore a Hippocratic oath should know better.

The reality is that over 30% of men respond poorly to these medications, and many men experience side effects that are quite undesirable. These side effects can range from nasal congestion, runny nose, headache, flushing, upset stomach, back pain, muscle pain, nausea, and dizziness. And in some cases, loss of vision, hearing impairment, or a priapism (an erection that lasts for more than 4 hours). While a 4-hour erection sounds like a night of awesome sex and bragging rights with your friends, the actual experience is much less favorable. For starters, most women are going to be rather sore and disinterested after 4 hours of sustained sex. The longer the erection lasts, the more likely serious physical complications can develop in your penis.

Now let's talk about heart problems and blood pressure. If you have heart problems or are on blood pressure medications, you may be at risk of a heart attack, stroke, irregular heartbeat, or drastic drop in blood pressure. While these are quite worrisome, they are also rare. It is your health practitioner's responsibility to take the time to gather your medical history, determine the root cause of your E.D., and evaluate your risks. Armed with this information, they can decide whether or not you are a candidate for these medications. It is perhaps only now that the full scope of possible negligence comes to light, especially when ordering these medications over the internet or from online clinics that don't perform a physical exam or thorough medical history.

I have seen thousands of E.D. patients and have heard countless stories of men experiencing these side effects. As there is an appropriate time and place for such a pill, I've had the unfortunate experience to witness this first-hand. One such event involved an elderly gentleman that neglected to inform me that he had recently added additional blood pressure meds from his cardiologist. One Saturday morning, he had the idea that if the usual dose of Viagra worked well, then a double-dose would work even better. When he didn't return from fetching the morning paper, his wife became worried and found that he had face-planted in the back yard after passing out from severely reduced blood pressure.

This unfortunate situation only helped to reinforce my approach of conducting a full and thorough intake, even though this gentleman had inadvertently withheld some information from me. Thank goodness he was not injured, other than his pride. These pills need to be taken seriously, not the stuff of stand-up comedy we have been led to believe. I do not take them lightly and nor should you. Then again, a pill might sound more appealing than the next treatment option.

TriMix Penile Injections

Yes, you did read that headline correctly. We are about to discuss an injection into your penis that is administered (by you) just before intercourse. This medication, called TriMix, is a mixture of three drugs (alprostadil, papaverine, and phentolamine). They work together to help vasodilate the blood vessels in the penis when the pills do not work or have undesirable side effects. While this does sound rather drastic, the medication is safe (when used correctly), has been in use since the mid-1980s, and produces positive results. We have about a 98% success rate with this option at our clinic. So, there is a time and place for it.

The challenge is that this medication must be carefully selected, and in some cases, custom blended to suit each patient. This involves administering a test dose in the clinic and then monitoring the penis to determine how quickly the erection forms, how firm it gets, and how long it lasts. Yes, you read that part right as well. There is indeed work that must be performed by a trained professional to get this right. Based on the results of the test dose, the physician recommends a specific formula and volume of medication that is self-administered via injection before intercourse. There is somewhat of an art form to get the dosage right, and if you visit a doctor that does not specialize in E.D., does not fully understand the medication, is not experienced in how to dose correctly, or do a thorough job of instructing you, the results can be undesirable or dangerous. Not to mention you've just allowed someone to monitor your erection with less than stellar results. It is also worth mentioning that some high-volume E.D. clinics use female nurses or Physician Assistants to perform the procedure.

While they may be professional, some men are very sensitive and embarrassed about allowing a female to perform the procedure.

There are also variations on this approach with BiMix and QuadMix, which offer options when Trimix is not effective. Another form of this approach is a topical/intraurethral gel called Muse®. The gel is inserted in the urethra with a special device and then massaged into the tissue of the urethra. I have found this option best suits very minor cases of E.D.; however, side effects may include a burning sensation in the urethra. All of these options are only effective for a one-time use and must be repeated before each sexual encounter. You must also wait at least 24 hours between each application. In addition, you must have a plan for addressing an accidental priapism (the persistent and painful 4-hour erection), which is also very important to keep you out of the hospital emergency room. So, does anyone want to give this treatment a try without a thorough intake from a knowledgeable physician who understands all of the risks? I didn't think so.

ED Rings (aka the Cock Ring)

When prescription medications are undesirable or work poorly, there is a possible solution for mild erectile dysfunction where a firm erection can be achieved initially, but then softens prematurely. In these cases, an E.D. ring may be a good option.

What is this medical mystery ring, you ask? These rings are placed around the base of the penis to prevent or slow the outflow of blood and make erections harder, bigger, and last longer. They come in different materials, from flexible silicone and rubber to leather, plastic, and even metal. They work best when a man can achieve a partial or full erection but has difficulty maintaining it.

The use of an E.D. ring can be a bit tricky as getting the device on and off can prove to be challenging. If you don't practice man-scaping, then you must be careful to avoid catching any hairs under the ring to prevent discomfort. In addition, some men report less powerful orgasms and difficulty ejaculating due to the pressure on the urethra from the ring. Removing the ring can also be challenging, depending on how tight it is, and if lubricant is used. Note that you must be careful not to fall asleep with the ring on as it may reduce healthy blood flow to the penis. One last caution for men with blood clotting disorders or men on blood thinners as these conditions should have the approval of a doctor before use. These rings can also be used in conjunction with a VED, as we will discuss in the next section.

VED (Vacuum Erection Device, aka The Penis Pump)

Often the source of humor, I am confident that you've heard about these devices. If you are a fan of the Austin Powers movies, you've seen Mike Meyers use one as a prop for a little penile humor. While some are sold as sex toys, you might be surprised to find that some are also developed legitimate medical devices to assist men experiencing E.D. In most cases, these are used when no other options are found to be effective.

The VED consists of a plastic cylinder that is placed over the penis with a seal at the base. Air is removed from the cylinder with either an electric pump or a manual pump. As the air is removed, blood is pulled into the penis until it is fully engorged. After this is done, a rubber restrictor-band (E.D. Ring) band is placed around the base of the penis to trap the blood in the penis. The cylinder is removed, and the "erect" penis can be used for intercourse.

While these may work well for some, there are negative aspects. These include the requirement to place the device on the penis prior to sex and maintaining sufficient firmness levels. They are prone to short duration erections from losing/leaking blood from the penis during sex, and the stiffness doesn't quite feel natural. Even with this negative discussion, these can be a viable solution when nothing else works. Much like the penile injections, there is a place for this treatment, just not one you may want to pursue when other options are available and preferable.

Penis Implants are a Real Thing

Finally, let's talk about one of the most extreme options available to us. Many men may not be aware of them, but the penis implant is actually a real thing. Implants are often associated with women and their breasts when it comes to enhancing sexual appearance and experience. With regard to men, it would be highly inadvisable to pursue a penis implant as an elective choice simply to enhance your appearance or experience. This path should only be pursued when all other options have failed, and you are not quite ready to give up on enjoying sex. The implant cannot be reversed, and only those men healthy enough to recover from a painful surgery should undergo the procedure. So, if you are in your 80's and just looking for a simple fix to be the sexual rock star of your retirement community, you are not a likely candidate.

This requires the use of a surgically implanted device, which becomes a permanent fixture of your body. Again, this option is reserved for cases when no other solution will work. In most cases, this is when the penile blood vessels, tissues, or nerves are severely damaged and will not respond to oral medications, Trimix injections, or a penis pump. The drawbacks of this solution include high expense, extensive surgery, and painful recovery. Without delving into in-depth detail, the three options for an implant include the following.

Three-piece inflatable - When inflated, a three-piece inflatable implant acts and feels the most like a natural erection. The implant also feels natural and comfortable when flaccid. In short, the implanted pumping device allows you to manually inflate and deflate your erection on command.

Two-piece inflatable - This is similar to the three-piece inflatable device and works similarly. The two-piece device is not as rigid as the three-piece implant. In some cases, the selection is a matter of preference, and in others, it is a matter of necessity.

Semi-rigid/malleable rods - This implant involves two flexible rods implanted into the penis. The implants don't change in size or stiffness and maintain a semi-rigid state. While easy to use, many men find the constant rigid state to be a bit uncomfortable.

As you can imagine, many men decide to call it quits with regards to traditional sexual intercourse rather than pursue this extreme option. That being said, if you find yourself in a season of life where decades of sexual performance lay ahead, know that this is an option for you. Moreover, many men find a place of peace with this option and go on to live a fulfilling sexual life with their partner. The choice will be yours but only do so after you have received the best medical advice possible. Education is key, and hopefully, I have helped you in that regard. As painful as these options may seem, the next option can truly be devastating.

Do Nothing and Hope for the Best

Often in life, we are faced with complex decisions where right and wrong are not always clear. It is probably safe to say that you never imagined being faced with the decision between a penis pump or a penile implant, but here we are, nonetheless. While right and wrong may be ambiguous, the evidence is clear that no decision may be more costly. No decision means that you have resigned yourself and your partner to miss out on months, years, or perhaps the rest of a lifetime of meaningful sexual fulfillment. My sincere hope for everyone reading this book is that you reject that option and start pursuing your own plan today.

Indeed, some minor cases of erectile dysfunction may very well find resolutions after time. This is particularly true if you have sustained a recent injury, are temporarily on a specific medication, or even embarked on a radical lifestyle makeover with diet weight loss. The downside to trying to wait this out is you may have wasted precious time. There is a final end date to the human sexual experience for everyone. Days and weeks lost matter. The other risk of doing nothing is that you delay the opportunity to rule out a more significant medical issue where erectile dysfunction may be an early warning sign that something more serious is wrong.

One also has to remember that the point at which a man begins to seek help for his erectile dysfunction often only comes after a long period of denial that is stacked on top of a long period of lackluster sexual performance. You may be content to wait it out and hope for the best, but your partner may not be able to do the same. Your decision directly affects them, or perhaps it is better to say that your indecision affects them. Many times, as long as they see you are trying, they will be more likely to offer you grace and love throughout the process.

Delaying treatment for erectile dysfunction can also worsen and deepen the psychological problems that may be driving the erectile dysfunction, to begin with. If depression is your primary driver, ask yourself if intimate sexual experiences with your partner would provide relief during a bout with depression. If you struggle with anxiety, would a prolonged absence from the bedroom cause your partner to equally withdraw or perhaps into the arms of another? Would addressing your problem with erectile dysfunction now give you confidence in the bedroom before you lose it completely?

There is so much to be gained by addressing this problem now and so much to lose by trying to wait it out. The last thing I would want for each and every one of you after reading this book is for you to do nothing. I'm confident in *The Man Plan,* and I know it can be a transformational experience in your life. I also know that doing nothing is fraught with peril. I'm pulling for you with every ounce of my being as I have been in this field for some time now, and I've seen what success looks like. You deserve success. So, now that we've covered some of the more conventional approaches let's cover some of the outside-the-box solutions that have been pursued and available to you.

CHAPTER 7

OUTSIDE-THE-BOX APPROACHES TO ERECTILE DYSFUNCTION

In the last chapter, on the conventional approaches to handling E.D., we were working primarily with quick fixes that didn't actually address the underlying cause of the dysfunction. In essence, these were Band-aids that merely helped (some of the time) to create an erection when needed. We all want to get back in the game as soon as possible but rarely do the conventional methods provide a long-term solution. The best approach would be to identify the underlying cause so that we can offer a long-term solution while also providing options to continue sexual activity in the short term. So here, we will cover some outside-the-box approaches to erectile dysfunction. It may very well be that you've heard about some of these before, and perhaps you have even tried some of these approaches. As part of a comprehensive treatment program, they can do a lot of good. Alone, and without proper guidance, they do not stand much chance against the power of erectile dysfunction.

Lifestyle Changes to Combat Erectile Dysfunction

The body is an amazing biological machine that knows exactly how to repair itself if we can simply provide an environment that is favorable to repair. Do not misunderstand this to assume that you can simply wait out your erectile dysfunction. We already covered the dangers of that in the last chapter. However, you can leverage your body's ability to heal itself in a thoughtful and intentional manner. For instance, if you cut or injure yourself with a traumatic injury, your body doesn't require you to provide a specific set of instructions on how to repair the wound. It just goes to work repairing the damage because that is what it is programmed to do.

As physicians, our goal to assist the effort by cleaning the wound to remove dirt or debris, relocate the ends of a broken bone, or surgically repair tissues that have been cut or torn. We may then be required to add things that assist the body in its job of repair. This may include the replacement of lost blood or plasma, an IV with nutrients like sodium, potassium, magnesium, calcium, or glucose. The body then simply needs rest and quality nutrients or food to complete the repair on its own. I know that it may sound like I might be over-simplifying the doctoring process, but the body is by far the most miraculous healer in all the history of medicine. Again, as doctors, our job is to identify the cause of the problem and help create an environment where the body can work its repair magic.

Unfortunately, from an early age, we have far too often pushed the body to work overtime and operate on less than ideal fuel. Think high sugar, poor quality fats, sodas, low water intake, excess animal protein combined with a lack of sufficient rest, exposure to environmental assaults such as smoking or vaping along with elevated stress. It amazes me that we wonder why our bodies do not perform like they are supposed to with all of this abuse. All these factors cause potential illnesses like hypertension, elevated cholesterol, and diabetes, leading to inflammatory conditions and, ultimately, vascular damage and the dreaded E.D.

Fortunately, the body is very forgiving and works extremely hard to operate optimally . . . for a while. As we age, the effects of our lifetime assault on the body begin to take its toll. The parts begin to wear prematurely, and the systems start to work less efficiently. In the case of E.D., the vessels in our penis begin to narrow and become less flexible, nerves become damaged, and we may lack certain nutrients needed for optimal performance. In addition, we may be under tremendous stress, which physiologically prevents the mind/desire from cooperating with the plumbing. So, let's talk about how you can help your body while we fight through the treatment process.

Diet is that dreaded four-letter word that no one really wants to talk about. You are already missing out on sexual intimacy, and now I might be telling you to let go of your favorite comfort foods? Say it isn't so! So, let's call it "food choice" instead. For most men experiencing E.D., food choice is a central element to long term repair, especially those afflicted with diabetes and obesity. I call it the "keystone" to optimal sexual function and general wellness. We need to eliminate the foods that create the damage and replace them with foods that actually promote repair and nourish the tissues. These nurturing foods include unprocessed, whole-foods like fresh vegetables, fruits, grains, nuts, and healthy oils like avocado and olive oil. Once again, you cannot "vegetable and fruit" your way out of erectile dysfunction. Gentlemen, I'm here to tell you that it helps more than you know. There is a beautiful cascade of events that occur when we get our food choices under control. I like to call it "pie-hole control." When we eliminate the poor foods and add healthy foods, then the following takes place.

When you eliminate poor quality food and eat health-promoting foods, your cholesterol will go down, and weight will drop. When your weight drops, your blood pressure falls, your blood sugar will normalize, and inflammation will be reduced. When that happens, you can reduce (dare I say eliminate) the medications that have been plaguing you. The body will be able to heal itself without unnecessary damage to blood vessels, kidneys, and nerves. Guess what happens next? **Your erections will improve**.

Again, we make the choices to take charge of our health with proper food selection, and the body has a fighting chance to repair the damage. Combine this with stress management in the form of more rest, meditation, exercise, and vacations for the win. Now, we have to understand that this doesn't happen overnight. The process takes time. We need to be consistent in our food selection, and even then, rebuilding and remodeling tissues take time. Think of how long it takes for the body to repair a cut or broken bone. The same thing is going on behind the scenes with the tissues and blood vessels in your penis. Be patient and be consistent. While you are working on this aspect of your life, we will explore other options to accelerate the process below.

Hormonal Adjustments to Fight Erectile Dysfunction

When it comes to diet and stress, most of you can easily speak the language. You've likely tried to diet before, and men in this modern era are unfortunately all too familiar with stress. So just a heads up that this next part is going to get a bit technical. I'll do my best to translate it into everyday language, but the world of hormones requires a little more technical jargon. Hormones come in many forms, and there are several that may be indirectly linked to erectile function. These include testosterone, Vitamin-D (yes, this is actually a hormone), and thyroid hormones.

Testosterone is indirectly linked to erections through libido/sexual desire. We know that testosterone production naturally drops as men age at about 1-2% per year. As testosterone wanes, so does our libido, which drives our desire for sex. Many people assume that low testosterone causes erectile dysfunction, but this is not necessarily true. The bottom line is that if we are not interested in sexual activities, then our likelihood of generating an erection diminishes. Remember that we have already discussed that the primary reason for E.D. in most men is insufficient blood flow due to vascular damage. With this in mind, correcting low testosterone levels will not likely resolve severe erectile dysfunction. It will help you want to have sex, but if the vascular damage is extensive, that want is not enough to "get it up."

Studies have also shown a correlation between E.D. and low Vitamin-D and low thyroid function (hypothyroid). Vitamin-D plays a vital role in many body functions. Research suggests that there is a correlation between adequate levels of vitamin D and adequate levels of testosterone. Vitamin-D is also linked to proper immune function, brain function, depression, blood sugar management, and cancer prevention through gene expression. While many think they get adequate Vitamin-D from the sun, studies indicate that many men are low and require oral supplementation, especially during the winter months. During the Winter months, cities above latitudes 42 deg N (i.e. Boston) do not get sufficient sunlight to make Vitamin-D. Even people in Southern cities such as Miami or Phoenix, are low in Vitamin-D because they spend less time outside and use more sunscreen. Other populations that may be at risk are African Americans, due to the melanin absorption, and obese patients.

Hypothyroidism can have an indirect effect on the hypothalamus and pituitary gland, thus interfering with testosterone production. Studies have found that 64% of men with hypothyroidism presented with low libido, erectile dysfunction, sperm abnormalities, and delayed ejaculation. *(The Journal of Clinical Endocrinology & Metabolism.* 1970;31(5):539-545.). It just makes sense to perform lab tests to determine if deficiencies in these areas are contributing to low testosterone and erectile dysfunction. That is why a thorough intake is essential to a real plan to fight erectile dysfunction. It is critical to have your doctor check your hormone levels to establish a baseline for your hormones.

Supplementation in the Fight Against Erectile Dysfunction

Essential nutrients also play a role in helping to curb erectile dysfunction. Keep in mind, this involves far more than just taking your daily Flintstone vitamins. The single most essential and fundamental molecule responsible for much of our erectile function is Nitric Oxide (NO). This is not to be confused with nitrous oxide (N_2O), the gas that dentists use to help us relax, and that race cars use for an extra boost. It would be nice if we could just take a boost of the stuff for a 'fast and furious' erection, but sadly, that is not the case. Nor is it Nitrogen Dioxide (NO_2), an environmental pollutant. Nitric Oxide is the miracle molecule that helps erections by dilating blood vessels when we are sexually aroused.

In addition, it helps the memory by transmitting information between nerve cells in the brain, assists the immune system with fighting off bacteria and defending against tumors. It regulates blood pressure by dilating arteries, reduces inflammation, and improves sleep quality. And finally, it increases your recognition of smell, improves athletic endurance, and assists gastric motility (moving food through the intestines). Like I said, it's a miracle molecule that does a lot.

For a number of reasons, our production of nitric oxide drops significantly by the time we are in our 60's. This may help to explain the subtle increase in both E.D. and blood pressure as we age. Increasing Nitric oxide can come from several sources, including:

- Vegetables high in nitrates such as Celery, Kale, Arugula, Lettuce, Beetroot, and Spinach

- Supplements with specific amino acids, such as L-arginine and L-citrulline

- Increased exercise, which improves the health of the inner wall of your blood vessels

- Limiting the use of mouthwash, which kills the beneficial bacteria on your tongue that help to produce nitric oxide

- Eliminating the use of fluoride in your toothpaste because fluoride kills the beneficial bacteria on your tongue that help create nitric oxide

- Limiting the use of antacids, because stomach acid is needed to product nitric oxide.

Deficiencies in nitric oxide are not limited to men as women may have deficiencies as well. That being said, men have exclusive rights to the erection, and you would do well to boost your nitric oxide levels. Your female partner can join you in this pursuit as she will experience a range of health benefits from doing so alongside you. Much like staying on a diet, it is much easier if you have a partner in crime, and if it works, she will also be the beneficiary of an upgraded erection. So make it a team effort for the ultimate win.

Shockwave/Acoustic-wave Therapy to Fight Erectile Dysfunction

Shockwave Therapy (aka Extracorporeal Shockwave Therapy - ESWT) is a relatively recent entrant to the E.D. toolkit in the last 5 to 10 years. Given the scope of the problem with erectile dysfunction, we will take all the allies we can get. Fortunately for men everywhere, it is proving to be a formidable force in the resurrection of poor erections. Don't be alarmed by the name, as there isn't an electrical shock involved in the process. So, no one will be plugging your 'little buddy' into a light socket.

Shockwave/Acoustic-wave therapy refers to a controlled impulse of energy from a handheld medical device directed through the tissues of the penis. This technology has been used successfully since the 1980s in the treatment of kidney stones. More recently, it has been used with musculoskeletal injuries, cellulite therapy, and now erectile dysfunction. Depending on the root cause of the E.D., and the level of severity, ESWT has been demonstrated to help remove the micro-plaque within blood vessels and trigger the growth of healthy new blood vessels in the penis. While the exact mechanism is not fully understood, it is thought to amplify growth factors and protein synthesis to stimulate collagen growth and tissue remodeling.

In essence, it helps to turn back the clock by remodeling the damaged and aging tissues of the penis to increase blood flow and provide better erections. The process does not impart any significant discomfort and requires about 20-30 minutes per treatment session. Depending on the underlying cause of the E.D. and severity, it may require 6 to 18 (or more) treatments to regain appreciable erectile functionality. Effects can last 2-4 years, depending on the health status of the patient. If you are a cigarette smoker, a diabetic with uncontrolled blood sugar, or are exposed to chronic stress leading to ongoing vascular damage, you may need more treatments, and the results may not last as long.

GAINSWave® has done a fantastic job of commercializing the process with a systematic approach to this E.D. therapy, which includes additional daily therapies and supplements. If you have sought treatment elsewhere in recent years, this may not have been presented as an option. *The Man Plan* was written with the latest treatment options in mind, and it is our aim to update it as science and technology reveal new possibilities. In some cases, PRP (platelet-rich plasma), stem cells, or exosome injections are used in conjunction with the shockwave therapy to further enhance results. So, let's make sure we cover that next.

PRP (Platelet Rich Plasma) in the Fight Against Erectile Dysfunction

Platelet rich plasma (PRP) therapy is the science of concentrating the platelets from a patient's own blood and injecting it into tissue to accelerate healing. Once again, using the power of your own body to heal itself. It can be used for injured tendons, ligaments, muscles, joints, scars, and yes, the penis. We also use it in cosmetic surgery and hair growth procedures to accelerate healing and promote growth. PRP is a natural source of special signaling molecules called growth factors and cytokines that help reduce inflammation and promote the healing of injured tissues. This is not a new therapy, as research has been around since the 1970s and put into practice with surgical procedures in the '80s.

Notable examples of PRP use in the public eye include Tiger Woods' knee injury, Hines Ward and Polamalu of the Pittsburgh Steelers before winning Super Bowl XLII, Major League Baseball pitchers Takashi Saito and Bartolo Colon, and professional basketball player Stephen Curry. Kim Kardashian has been documented using PRP in a popular therapy called the Vampire Facelift® to help reduce the signs of aging on her face. There have been many examples where it has been used to treat erectile dysfunction, but those are less public. Let's face it, you don't hear too many male celebrities bragging about their inability to get an erection.

With regard to erectile dysfunction, PRP was popularized with a treatment called the P-Shot® (aka Priapus-Shot®, PRP-Shot) to help

83

men suffering from E.D. The PRP from your own blood is painlessly injected into targeted areas of the penis to initiate healing. The PRP promotes reduced inflammation, the growth of new blood vessels, improved circulation, increased penis girth, and size, for longer-lasting erections and more powerful orgasms. I have performed hundreds of these treatments with fantastic results. This is also a great add-on with the use of shockwave therapy to help increase favorable results. It is important to note that optimal results are also dependent on having optimized hormone levels. Smoking, diabetes, and other inflammatory conditions may also hinder the best outcome.

Stem Cells and Exosomes

You have probably noticed the increased press surrounding the recent use of stem cell therapy for a number of medical conditions. There are some profiteering companies spinning it as the new "snake oil," but don't let that distract you from the science. Stem cell therapy is real, and when wielded by proper medical practitioners, it holds a great deal of potential. Mesenchymal stem cells (MSC's), also known as Medicinal signaling cells, are potent cells found in various places in the body that can differentiate into various cell types for tissue repair. The stem cells work much like the PRP, in that they help repair damaged tissue, promote the growth of new and healthy tissue and blood vessels to promote better erections.

The most common method of harvesting one's own stem cells is adipose tissue-derived stem cells (ADSCs) and bone marrow-derived stem cells (BMSCs).   ADSCs are commonly collected using a minimally invasive technique very similar to liposuction.   BMSC is typically harvested from bone marrow from the hip bone. Both of these are relatively quick and safe, with minimal to moderate pain. Once the cellular material is collected, the MSC's are separated from the non-useful tissue and injected into the penis, much like the PRP.

Exosomes are an emerging new therapy for erectile dysfunction, which can be derived from stem cells. While stem cells have been the main focus for advanced regeneration of damaged tissues and disease for many years, we are now better understanding this new type of cellular material derived from young, healthy, Mesenchymal Stem Cells to jumpstart the healing process. Discovered over 50 years ago, exosomes are described as extracellular microvesicles (1/1000 the size of cells) that contain genetic information and proteins that are used as signaling agents for cell-to-cell communication in response to injuries.

In short, exosomes are the messengers that tell the older cells how and when to react in damaged tissues. Recent developments from leading companies in exosome research have shown great promise with effective protocols in treating erectile dysfunction and a number of other pathologies. Because of the biologic nature of exosomes, they can be derived from the cells of other healthy donors and concentrated for use in other people with little concern for cellular rejection or injury. If you could not quite follow the medical jargon, I apologize, but let's just sum it up to say that it is all good news for you and your penis.

Peptides versus Erectile Dysfunction

In my constant quest for additional therapies to help combat the battle with E.D., I've found a safe and promising treatment that uses an all-natural biological molecule called peptides. Peptides are not new, although new peptides are being discovered all the time. They are short chains of amino acids (2 to 50), which are the building blocks of proteins. In the human body, peptides are found in every tissue to perform a wide range of essential biologic functions. This includes the formation of hormones like insulin, prolactin, oxytocin, leptin, and growth hormone.

In particular, one peptide called Bremelanotide (aka PT-141) has been found to promote increased erectile activity in men with and without erectile dysfunction. Based on the dosage and severity of E.D., response time can range from minutes to several hours. Currently, PT-141 is administered via a simple injection in the waistline area. It must be noted that this is not a cure but rather a use-as-needed solution. However, if you are unwilling to cede days, weeks, months, and years of healthy sexual activity while you pursue a cure, these peptides may keep you active in the bedroom in the meantime.

Emotional Counseling/Psychological Therapy

We've discussed several biological factors and treatments for erectile dysfunction in this chapter. So, let's swing back around and make sure we cover a few psychological factors as well. As discussed earlier in this book, brain cooperation is the primary starting point in initiating an erection. There are a number of mental factors that can provide to be an obstacle to an erection, and that extends far beyond accidentally seeing a picture of your grandmother naked. These include stress (PTSD), anxiety, depression, relationship problems, childhood trauma, and even fear of sexual dysfunction.

I have found that some men respond well with particular treatments, only to discover later that E.D. challenges resurface sporadically. This may be indicative of emotional/psychological issues and requires time with the patient to help determine any underlying challenges that are not structural. This is just another important reason to find the right doctor who can establish a comfortable and trusting environment that allows you to open up to discuss an uncomfortable subject matter. Once you can better understand the underlying emotional triggers, it is easier to recommend an appropriate therapy. Possible therapies may include the following:

- Licensed Sex Therapist - Sex therapy is intended to help individuals and couples resolve sexual difficulties, such as performance anxiety and relationship problems. Clients usually meet in the therapist's office, and in some cases use telemedicine. Some choose to attend sessions alone; others bring their partner with them. Please note this is not just about having "better" sex. There are deep issues that some couples face, and you would do well to address them with a professional.

- Neuro Emotional Technique (NET) - is a proven blend of the latest scientific research and centuries-old Eastern healing techniques. NET addresses the relationship between the body's emotional health, environmental toxicity, nutritional balance, and structural integrity. It is a technique used to normalize unresolved physical and/or behavioral patterns in the body.

- Homeopathy - Long term emotional problems such as depression, chronic anxiety, PMS, sexual abuse, and lack of confidence may be addressed with constitutional homeopathy. This requires the skill of a well-trained homeopathic practitioner who will interview the individual to find the correct remedy out of the hundreds, which fits the pattern of symptoms expressed by the person. The remedy stimulates the body and mind to begin to heal on a deep cellular level. The result is a very profound yet gradual improvement. The emotional state becomes brighter, energy and vitality increase, and undesirable physical symptoms lessen.

In Summary

As you can see, there are a host of options available to you, and with the right instruction, they can really make a difference for you and your partner in the bedroom. Again, you may not have followed all the medical talk, but good news for you and your penis is the best summary. That's what makes me so frustrated when doctors instantly prescribe a pill without considering all the options. Erectile dysfunction is so much more complicated than that. While I don't throw the term around lightly, it feels almost negligent for some in the medical field to be so dismissive of other options. But you are here now, and you found me. I'm grateful for you making it this far in the book, and your partner will be proud of how much effort you are putting into fixing this problem. Stick with me just a little longer, and we'll be well on our way to the solution that you and your partner deserve.

CHAPTER 8

PEYRONIE'S DISEASE AND ERECTILE DYSFUNCTION

While we think of Erectile dysfunction as the general inability to generate an erection suitable for sexual activity, there is another less common form of E.D. that can be challenging to treat. This condition is called Peyronie's disease (pay-roe-NEEZ) and can prevent sexual activity due to a malformation in the tissues of the penis (a bend), making penetration remarkably difficult, or so painful that it is undesirable. That's the brief executive summary and perhaps how it is best well known. We're not talking a subtle one or two degrees off center, but a noticeable bend in the penis that often causes severe pain with an erection and inhibits sexual function. For many men reading this book, this is the primary reason that brought you here, and I'm sorry to have you wait until near the end of the book to address it in detail. Let me reassure you that all the previous chapters are still applicable to your struggle. Peyronie's disease is not mutually exclusive to all the other drivers of erectile dysfunction. You can suffer from Peyronie's disease and also be affected by vascular issues. You can have a drastic bend in your penis and suffer from anxiety, depression, or trauma.

Before we proceed with this chapter, let's address the elephant in the room. As a medical professional in this field for some time now, I realize how embarrassing this topic can be to discuss. You would not be the first man to break down into tears as you recount the traumatic sexual encounters and shame that you have been made to feel as a result of this condition. So, I'm going to encourage you to let down your guard a bit so that we can have a fruitful and meaningful conversation about what you are facing. It's just us men here talking, apart from the occasional woman reading this book to support her partner. Men, if you have a lady who is doing that for you, then she's a keeper. So, we'll allow her to be here too. The good news is that Peyronie's disease is treatable. Those same men who broke down in my office nearly broke down again when they realized that their traumatic journey had come to an end. There was always hope for them, but they just didn't know it. So it is with you today. There is hope in the battle against Peyronie's disease, and you are about to become a believer.

What is Peyronie's Disease

While it may be known as the curved penis disease, there is certainly a great deal more science and biology behind it. For starters, is Peyronie's Disease (P.D.) actually a disease? Not really, it is actually a physical condition of the penis named for François Gigot de la

Peyronie, a French surgeon (1678 – 1747) who described it in 1743. Specifically, Peyronie's disease results from fibrous scar tissue that develops in the penis. The symptoms of the disease may come about quickly, or they may gradually develop over a long time. It is known as the curved penis disease because that is one of the most common and obvious developments. The penis may curve upward or downward or to one side or the other. Again, this is not just a few degrees off-center or the Leaning Tower of Pisa. If you have a significant curve, there is no mistaking it.

The other symptoms may be less known, but equally damaging to man's ability to sexually perform at the desired level. So let's talk about the scar tissue itself. Scar tissue associated with Peyronie's disease is known as plaque. Not to be confused with the plaque that can build up in your blood vessels or the plaque that can develop on your teeth, this plaque is the source of what ails you. As it develops, you may feel the plaque under the skin of the penis in either flat lumps or perhaps a band of hard tissue. If you think that you may be developing this and have yet to be diagnosed with Peyronie's disease, it would be good to schedule a visit with a qualified medical practitioner. This is particularly true if you are also suffering from erectile dysfunction.

Erection problems can be an early indicator of Peyronie's disease. Men will often notice the trouble with the erection long before seeing other symptoms of Peyronie's. Pain is another symptom that often drives men to seek help. This penile pain can be with or without an erection. In general, your penis should not be causing you pain for any given reason. After all, it should be the fun factory and not the pain factory. So if you are experiencing penile pain, please seek medical advice. In some cases, Peyronie's disease may cause a range of other penile deformities. This could be narrowing indentations and even an hourglass looking shape with a tight, narrow band around the shaft. Once again, if you see it, you know that this is not normal.

This brings us to the final symptom of Peyronie's and one that many men dread. Peyronie's disease can also cause a shortening of the penis. That's right, men, the penis can go in the opposite direction that both you and your partner would preference. If left untreated, the curvature and the shortening can worsen over time. Though it will typically stabilize within the first year. However, if six months to a year penis shortening sounds less than helpful to you, then it is time to take action. The pain may subside in a couple of years, but the curvature or shortening will remain if left untreated. The earlier the intervention, the better chances you have in the fight against Peyronie's. Now that you know what it is let's talk about what causes it.

Causes of Peyronie's Disease

A singular cause of Peyronie's disease is not always clear or even thoroughly understood. That's why a one-stop solution for all men simply does not work. There are, however, several common factors involved that we could explore. The first and often most commonly assumed is repeated or significant injury to the penis. The penis can become damaged in a variety of ways, one of which would be the "breaking" of the penis during sexual intercourse. Yes, gentlemen, you can break your penis, and there is no confusion about the matter when it happens. Obviously, there is no actual breaking of a bone of any sort. However, in the heat of passion, a man can "miss the target," resulting in his penis impacting with great speed and force against an impenetrable part of his partner. In some instances, a very noticeable "pop" can be felt. It is typically followed by an intense feeling of pain with screeching and yelling. Fellas, this is not the type of moaning one would hope for during intercourse.

Another way the penis could become damaged is through athletic activity or any other accident where trauma is induced upon the penis. As the body begins to heal itself, the scar tissue begins to develop. The only problem is that for many men, the scar tissue does not form in any organized fashion. The scar or nodules that you can feel under the skin eventually cause the curvature of the penis. Subsequently, when blood flows to the penis during an erection, the rest of the penis stretches while the scar tissue does not. The result is a disfigured and painful erection. While some trauma to the penis is most commonly assumed, you may be surprised to find out that most report no known injury to the penis before suffering from Peyronie's.

This sends us back to square one and leaves us to examine other risk factors. One's own genes can be a contributing factor for Peyronie's disease. If you have had a family member suffer from Peyronie's, you now have an increased risk of the condition. While we know this to be true, it is quite challenging to assess. The reality is that not too many fathers or grandfathers share the story of their curved penis with their offspring. It could be a contributing factor to you right now, but you simply do not know it. If you dare to ask your father if he has a straight penis or not, then good for you. Most men are, unfortunately, left guessing.

Connective tissue disorders can also be a driver of the disease. Men who struggle with some connective tissue disorders appear more likely to have an increased risk of developing Peyronie's. In addition, we know that age is a risk factor, as well. Men in their 50's and 60's are known to suffer more from the disease. Just as men in that age range struggle more with other factors of erectile dysfunction, it seems to be the case here as well. Younger men who have not experienced penile trauma may experience curvature of the penis, but this is mostly known as congenital penile curvature. If you are a younger man and are simply a little off-center, do not worry as this is entirely normal.

Certain types of prostate surgery, smoking, and other health conditions can be contributing factors as well. The truth is that apart from known and obvious trauma, it is not always clear why a man suffers from this disease. Fortunately, there are treatment options available for most men. Beyond just painful erections, Peyronie's disease can cause men to have anxiety and stress about having sexual intercourse, further contributing to erectile dysfunction. It can add a great deal of stress to your relationship, and if that wasn't bad enough, it can shorten your penis. So, with that being said, most men should be ready to hear about the treatment options. Without further ado, let's start solving the problem.

Treatment Options of Peyronie's Disease

Once you've sought help for what you believe to be Peyronie's disease, the diagnosis can come fairly quickly. Often a physical exam where the doctor will examine your penis when it is not erect can identify the location and the amount of scar tissue involved. They might even measure your penis to get some data to evaluate if the condition is worsening or stabilized. There could also be a scenario where your doctor may ask you to bring a picture of your erect penis. This may seem odd at first, but trust me, it is perfectly normal and part of the analysis.

You may be asked to schedule an ultrasound or get an MRI. You may also receive an injection into your penis that causes it to be erect for better evaluation. This is quite helpful as it will allow the physician to visualize the deformity and palpate the areas in question. From there, the key is to try to determine whether you are in the acute phase or the chronic phase. The acute phase is what you would identify first and early on into the struggle. Typically, this would be in the first month or so when you notice symptoms but could stretch into the first year. The chronic phase is when the damage is done, so to speak. You may not have continued pain, and the advancement in curvature or deformity seems to be over. Depending on what phase you are in will determine the course of action. So let's run through some of the options that we might order.

Medications - This treatment regimen may include oral medication, injections, or some combination thereof. The notion of receiving an injection into your penis may sound painful, but in many cases, you will get a local anesthetic. One of the medications that may be used is collagenase. Known as collagenase clostridium histolyticum, this is actually the only FDA-approved medication. This medication is quite expensive but has proven to produce improvements in curvature and other troubling symptoms. It may also be combined with "modeling," which is a forced bending of the penis in the opposite direction to help induce straightening. Also, note that this medication can also cause severe damage to the penis if administered by someone other than a trained and skilled medical practitioner. Other drugs such as Verapamil, which has historically been used to treat high blood pressure and cardiac conditions, and Interferon have been observed to hold potential as well. Verapamil targets the production of collagen, while Interferon targets the production of fibrous tissue.

Traction Therapy - Needless to say, any treatment for Peyronie's disease is often less than pleasant. However, if you are dedicated to a healthy sexual future, then you must be willing to go the distance. Penile traction therapy involves stretching the penis with a mechanical device. Now, this might seem like Medieval torture, and in some cases, you would be correct. However, safely applied, this therapy holds the potential to improve the length, deformity, or curvature. In some cases, you would wear it for an hour or less, while in other cases, a full 8-hour workday would be necessary. This therapy is most often used early on in the treatment phase. It is uncomfortable, but as they say in the military, an ounce of sweat today will save you a gallon of blood tomorrow. So, in this case, a little discomfort today may save you a gallon of penile pain tomorrow.

Surgery - Now, no one likes the thought of having surgery on the penis, but you also may not enjoy the idea of living with a deformed penis forever. This option is typically reserved for the more severe cases where you are unable to have sex due to the pain and deformity. It may also seem counter-intuitive since the very act of performing surgery is going to leave scar tissue in the penis. In extreme cases, a penile implant may be utilized. This is not the preferred course, but an implant can be inserted into the spongy tissue that fills with blood during an erection to straighten the penis. At the end of the day, only a qualified medical professional can identify what type of surgery is needed. However, I would recommend that you walk into that appointment armed with all the information available. All doctors take the same Hippocratic oath, but sadly, not all doctors are equal. So "do no harm" always applies, but "do no harm" to the penis should be emphasized with greater importance.

Alternative Treatments - Beyond the treatments mentioned above, science and medicine are frequently looking for more alternatives to treat Peyronie's disease. It is not that these treatments are speculative or do not show promise, but the results are often mixed. However, for a man at the end of his rope looking for a solution, they can be impactful and always worth evaluation. One such technique is known as iontophoresis. This is where an electric current is used to administer a combination of verapamil and a steroid through the skin. The results are mixed, but some show improvement in erectile function as well as the curvature of the penis. Another non-drug, non-surgical treatments that I have performed involves the use of focused ESWT (extracorporal shockwave therapy). We discussed shockwave therapy earlier, although, in this application, it serves to help break up the scar tissue. When combined with platelet-rich plasma, stem cells, and a VED device, I have seen this successfully straighten the penis over time. It may be that one of these options is right for you, but the only way to know is to seek help. If your doctor did not mention or was not aware of these possibilities, then they perhaps did not serve you best. Bring them up and at least enter them into the discussion.

A Conclusion of Hope

At the end of the day, what is right for you may not be right for another man. Yet, what you both have is hope. The inability to treat Peyronie's disease in some fashion is rare. There need not be any man who is permanently affected by this disease before trying all the options. I know that this disease has likely caused you physical pain and mental trauma. Just know that you are not alone. This disease has come upon you through no fault of your own, but through dedication and a willingness to seek help, it will cease to be the burden you have known it to be. Peyronie's disease, just like every cause of erectile dysfunction, can be beaten. It will require a thorough intake, and most importantly, any solution requires you to address the root cause. That is the silver bullet, and anything short of addressing the root causes and primary drivers will not do. That is what we will discuss in the next chapter, and you are one step closer to a solution and a future of healthy sexual activity.

CHAPTER 9

THE ULTIMATE SOLUTION: ADDRESSING THE ROOT CAUSE

Here we are in Chapter 9, and sadly, you have already done more research and assessment on erectile dysfunction than many of the medical practitioners out there promising a quick fix. At the end of the day, this your penis. There may be many like it, but this one is yours. Few people will care more about your penis than you, and you have to be the biggest advocate for it. Maybe your partner will join in the advocacy, but you get the point. You simply can't assume that because someone has the title "doctor" or "nurse," they will give you the time and attention you deserve.

I should also warn you about the profit motive. There are a number of expensive new treatments that have surfaced in the last several years that may not help everyone, despite what a doctor or his sales staff may say. With the advent of generic Viagra and Cialis and these expensive treatment protocols, there has been an increase in the number of doctors "specializing" in men's sexual wellness. The sad reality is that many of these doctors and clinics don't take the time to adequately address your situation and are merely chasing the money through a few quick and easy treatment options. Your penis has done you a lot of good over the years, so please take the time to find the right provider who cares as much as you.

As you've found while reading this book, there are a multitude of systems that can go awry in the human-machine to cause E.D.. These include the brain, the nervous system, your hormones, and the vascular system, for a multitude of reasons. Despite any popular new therapy that a doctor might be pushing, there is simply no "one-size-fits-all" solution for erectile dysfunction. If you walk into a doctor's office for erectile dysfunction seeking answers and walk out with a prescription in less than 15-30 minutes without a thorough understanding, then you have been to the wrong clinic. It's either a thorough intake or bust in my book. So let's talk about the intake.

Digging Deep for the Root Cause

Your doctor cannot read your mind, and it is imperative for your doctor to understand all aspects of your background. We need to go over the detailed circumstances of your current situation and how long erectile dysfunction has been present. I want to hear about what therapies you have tried and even how committed your partner is to seeking a solution and being a part of the process. If it is part of your medical or social history, then I want to know about it. Yet, even with a full medical history, it often turns out to be the most obscure piece of information that solves the puzzle.

I have had men with no apparent past medical problems arrive with erectile dysfunction that seemingly cannot be explained. Only after thorough questioning about even the most benign OTC medications for seasonal allergies does the actual cause surface. Believe it or not, taking allergy meds can be a recipe for erectile disaster. In particular, some decongestant medications taken to prevent a runny nose can be the simple cause of your erectile dysfunction. Often, these medications aren't mentioned because they aren't used daily. Few men would ever connect their seasonal allergies with their E.D. That's why a thorough intake can save the patients substantial money on unnecessary E.D. medications or therapies.

A Blast from the Past Case Study - One particular patient in his early 40s came to my clinic accompanied by his girlfriend and expressed that he had never achieved a full erection in his life. This is probably a fact his girlfriend would have liked to have known before entering into a relationship with him, but no one really shares that on a first date. He had been to several urologists that were unable to determine the root cause of his E.D. and find a suitable solution other than a penis implant. He stated that he did not respond to high doses of Viagra or Cialis in the past and was in despair.

I pulled out all of my medical books and diagrams and guided him through the entire cascade of neurologic and biological events required to generate an erection. This included emotional issues, physical trauma, medications, and even environmental chemical exposures that he may have encountered in his youth. When nothing seemed to fit, I asked him to dig deep in his memory for anything in his past that might correlate to what he had just seen and heard. He brought up a seemingly unrelated story that happened when he was about 10 years old. He and a buddy had rebuilt a bicycle from spare parts and were ready to take it for a test ride.

He volunteered for the job, and as he was pedaling as fast and hard as possible, the chain came off, and he came down and slammed his groin into the top tube of the frame so hard that he passed out from the pain. In today's day and age, such a video would have gone viral, but this was before the ubiquitous cell phone camera. He vaguely remembered being black and blue and having numbness in the groin area for some time. That's it. That's all he knew.

Yet, with this information, we were able to pinpoint the trauma that damaged the nerves that provided the signal to his penis to trigger an erection. Without this signal, there is little stimulus to the penis to initiate an erection, and medications like Cialis will not be effective. We were able to perform a test dose with Trimix and induce the first quality erection that he had experienced in his life. Needless to say, he and his girlfriend were in tears of joy and pleased with the results.

Sorting Through the Variables

If a bicycle accident at the age of 10 can cause 30 years of erectile dysfunction, then what else could you and your doctor be missing? That's why we have to sort through all the variables. Family history may lead to information about the potential for prostate issues, diabetes, high blood pressure, or vascular diseases. Meanwhile, understanding social history is another crucial area that must be addressed. Exercise, energy level, employment, home situation, alcohol consumption, smoking, drug use, and even emotional abuse need to be evaluated.

The emotional history includes their basic nature/disposition, worries, fears, depression, anxiety, or any previous diagnosis of mental or emotional disorders. This ties back to the need to have our nervous system in a parasympathetic state or mood. If we are constantly worrying or have anxiety, it makes it increasingly challenging to generate an erection. Coupled with this, we need to ask if any medications are being used to combat anxiety or depression that could be a contributing factor.

Diet can play a central role in how you developed erectile dysfunction. As we discussed, obesity and Type 2 diabetes typically develop as a result of diet issues, which leads to vascular inflammation and, ultimately, atherosclerosis and E.D.. Do you drink excessive caffeinated products like coffee, soda, or energy drinks? This can lead to nervous anxiety and put your nervous system in a "fight or flight" state that may contribute to erectile dysfunction. Sleep is another essential factor, as we "recharge" our batteries when sleeping, which includes cortisol (our stress hormone), and testosterone. I see patients that work night shift (firemen, policemen, factory workers) who have issues with low testosterone, adrenal fatigue, and low energy, all having an impact on optimal sexual

DR. DAN LARKE

performance. Insomnia and sleep apnea can also contribute to the problem.

Did your doctor cover all the factors above? Or did they reach for the pen after a 10-minute conversation to write a prescription? Sadly, doctors often even take shortcuts with the basic physical exam. This should include examining blood pressure and a basic check of the heart and lung sounds. The physician should perform a thorough examination of the pelvic area and genitalia. Honestly, you would think that this is the first place they would look, but you would be surprised. They should be observing any deformities or scarring in the penis, plaque formation, scrotal masses, urethral discharges, or any abnormalities under an existing foreskin. Any testicular abnormalities may indicate possible testicular cancer.

Any active Herpes sores or history of herpes should be brought to the physician's attention as well as venereal warts such as HPV (herpes papillomavirus). Though this doesn't necessarily cause E.D., although it may contribute to performance anxiety if you are just starting to become sexually active with a new partner. Any pain or tenderness noted during the examination should be brought to the doctor's attention as it may provide clues to the underlying issues. Advanced diagnostic testing and evaluation may include blood hormone testing and the use of ultrasound to provide a general condition of blood flow through the penile tissues. In some cases, it may be appropriate to give a Trimix injection to evaluate the penis

106

in the erect state. This may help diagnose Peyronie's disease or a venous leak, which may not otherwise have been observed.

Addressing the Root Cause

I want to quickly clarify that addressing the root cause does not mean delaying any form of relief until the "perfect" solution is discovered. Whether the root cause is physical or psychological, a quick and easy, <u>short-term solution</u> can be provided to keep you in action until a long term solution can be provided. Truth be told, I do have patients that are simply not interested in a long term solution, but rather just want something to help them today. This can be in the form of PD5E-inhibitors (Viagra, Cialis), Trimix, or even peptides. We must remind ourselves that these are just "band-aid" solutions to generate an erection today, and don't address the root cause of the problem.

Just be aware that a high percentage of men with severe E.D. simply don't respond well to the PD5E-inhibitors and may cause uncomfortable side effects. In my years of practice, I have seen a very high success rate with the Trimix. However, not all men are comfortable administering an injection to the side of their penis before every sexual encounter.

So I get it. An erection today is worth more than a hypothetical erection tomorrow. I'm not opposed to helping you find sexual fulfillment while addressing the broader issues, but your penis needs you to be all-in on a long-term solution if that's what you really want.

A Diet and Lifestyle Case Study - One of my new patients in his mid-30's came to my office in despair over the fact that he was experiencing E.D. at such an early age. He was happily married with 2 children and didn't see this coming. Moreover, he was 6 feet 5 inches tall and a former collegiate basketball athlete. However, he was now classified as obese and battling pre-diabetes along with his wife. It would have been easy to simply pull out my Rx pad and write a prescription for Viagra or Cialis, but it was my duty as a physician to help him understand the root cause.

You see, his dilemma was likely his diet and lifestyle, which led to obesity and diabetes. One of the principles I learned in medical school that really resonated with me was the Latin term "Docere," which translates to "Doctor as teacher." With this in mind, when the patient is willing to listen, it is incumbent on me to take the time to teach them about their disease. Long term, this helps them to learn and prevent it from returning in the future. In this case, he was interested in learning, so I taught.

I went into detail about the physiology of diabetes, how it leads to vascular damage, and directed him to some books to read, and a movie to watch. As excited as I was to help him, he never came back for a follow-up appointment. I had actually forgotten about him until the day he walked back into the office about 6 months later and gave me a big bear hug to say thank you for our talk.

He explained that he had gone home after our visit and watched the documentary I recommended (Forks Over Knives) with his wife and children. He said that movie changed his life as he and his wife both went on to lose over 40 pounds each and regain their health and his sexual function. He has subsequently adopted the new diet and lifestyle for his entire family. In this case, he had a mild form of diabetes, and he made changes early enough to correct his health in a relatively short amount of time.

A Combined Approach

I think one of my biggest problems with some of my peers in the field is the short-sighted approach. It just doesn't have to be that way. You can seek a short-term erection and a long-term solution. Not only is there not a one size fits all solution, but often the answer is actually multiple solutions. It is important to note that the positive, long-term results of some therapies are dependent on reducing obesity, diabetes, smoking, chronic stress, high blood pressure, and high cholesterol. As we discussed, the inflammation from these illnesses causes ongoing vascular damage. If we allow these to progress unchecked, then other treatments will be compromised and not be as effective. Here are a few different solutions that may be one part of a combined approach that should only be pursued after gaining complete understanding from a thorough intake.

ESWT (Extracorporeal Shockwave Therapy) - This is a solution that can be explored to accelerate the repair of vascular damage in the penis and pelvic area. As discussed earlier in the book, this involves weekly treatments with an FDA approved device to impart impulse/shock/acoustic waves through the targeted tissues to help remodel them and grow new, healthy blood vessels. Again, this is not an instant fix. We are merely encouraging the body to repair the damaged tissue a bit faster than normal. GAINSWave® has done a lot of work to promote this approach, which combines other therapies such as the VED (vacuum erectile device) in their protocol.

PRP (platelet-rich plasma) - This was popularized with a treatment called the P-Shot® (aka Priapus-Shot®, PRP-Shot) to help men suffering from mild E.D. The PRP from your own blood is painlessly injected into specific areas of the penis to initiate healing. PRP helps to promote reduced inflammation, the growth of new blood vessels, improved circulation, increased penis girth and size, longer lasting erections, and more powerful orgasms. I have performed hundreds of these treatments with fantastic results. This is also a great add-on with the use of shockwave therapy to provide synergistic results. It is important to note that optimal results usually take weeks (even months) to see and are also dependent on having optimized hormone levels. Moreover, diet, smoking, diabetes, and other inflammatory conditions may hinder the best outcome if not concurrently addressed.

Stem Cells and Exosomes - We covered these in past chapters and noted that MSC stem cells from your own body or donor tissues can be used to help the body repair/remodel damaged erectile tissues, including blood vessels and nerves. Again, It is important to note that optimal results usually take many weeks to develop and are dependent on having optimized hormone levels. Once again, diet, smoking, diabetes, and other inflammatory conditions have an effect. Are you starting to see the pattern? Regardless of what others have told you, multiple issues are likely driving your E.D., and that is why a combined approach is often so effective.

Mental/Emotional/Psychological - Some of this can be accomplished in the office with discussions that simply bring particular life stressors into the light. In most cases, this requires the help of a trained professional counselor to understand the nuances of the circumstances that have caused the E.D.. On a positive note, many of the "quick fix" remedies work wonderfully to help achieve an erection until the challenges can be addressed with the counselor. It is always a good idea to explore hormone testing and review the diet to ensure that all systems are working optimally.

A Final Plea for a Thorough Intake

Medical professionals have to cover it all. Perhaps I should rephrase that. I have to cover it all because I know too much and I care too much. I refuse to take the easy route when I know you and your partner deserve more. You simply cannot come to the right conclusion and course of treatment from a 2-minute questionnaire. A pill may get you a decent erection today, but it will do nothing for the continued despair that you are building up for yourself and your partner tomorrow. As I said before, it's a thorough intake or bust in my book. Literally, this is my book, and I'll promote nothing less. It is my sincere hope that you are ready for the change you deserve, but before I ask you to take the next step on your journey, we'll wrap this conversation up nicely.

CHAPTER 10

ONE STEP AWAY FROM THE ROCKSTAR ERECTION YOU DESERVE

In 2014, Navy Admiral William H. McRaven gave a commencement speech to the University of Texas and offered perhaps the most practical advice for tackling the most significant problems in our lives. Speaking of the elite Navy SEAL regimen, Admiral McRaven told graduates that if they wanted to change the world, it all started with making their beds in the morning. He went on to explain that when you make your bed, you have accomplished the first task of the day. It will give you an early sense of pride in your day, and it will encourage you to accomplish another task and then another.

Now, I'm not sure whether you have made your bed this morning, but you are about to finish this book. That means if you have been plagued by erectile dysfunction for any period of time, you are about to accomplish the first task on your road to recovering the rockstar erections that you deserve. You should be filled with a sense of pride that inspires you to take the next steps on the road to recovery. I'm excited for you right now. Your partner should be excited for you and for themselves. Most importantly, you should be excited because your struggle is about to become a thing of the past.

A Brief Review of Erectile Dysfunction

We won't delay your recovery by having you read the book again in the final chapter, but it would be a good idea to summarize much of what we have learned. Doing so will empower you with the information you need to take this much crucial next step. First of all, remember what brought you to this book in the first place.

My partner gave me an ultimatum - If that is what brought you there, then congratulations. Tell your partner that they have been heard, and you are ready for a new life.

My partner thinks that I don't love them or find them attractive - Go to your partner right now and tell them that they are beautiful, stunning, and the object of your affection. Encourage them that a new day is around the corner.

I can't keep a partner because I ejaculate so quickly - Well, you may or may not be able to get one of the old one's back. However, you can start courting the new apple of your eye, knowing that the next time you head to the bedroom, it won't be a quick trip back home.

My partner says they are ok with my E.D., but I know that's not true - This is the point where you tell them that you know they were lying for your sake, but it's ok. A new day is dawning for both of you in the bedroom.

Whatever it was that brought you, be encouraged. You are one step away from the recovery process. Remember what brought you here and let that fuel you on to take the next step with speed and intensity. You both deserve it.

Sexual Dysfunction Can be Treated

Remember that for nearly every case of sexual dysfunction, there is an answer. Are you struggling with low libido? We can examine that and find a path forward. Erectile dysfunction throwing a curve in your romantic relationships? There is a solution. Is a curve in your penis throwing a curve in your relationship? There is a plan for that too. Sexual dysfunction takes on many forms, and The Man Plan is a plan to combat them all.

This plan takes into account the full spectrum of primary drivers of erectile dysfunction and its risk factors. It targets the vascular network in your penis to ensure it is functioning at an optimal level. Neurological factors caused by events like prostate surgery or spinal injuries will be explored. We'll take a review of your medications and see if the fix for one ailment is the cause of another. You'll have the opportunity to examine your lifestyle in detail to determine if there may be daily factors driving your inability to produce a strong and powerful erection.

We'll also take a deep dive into the emotional side of erectile dysfunction. Anxiety, depression, lack of confidence all play a role. If needed, we'll recommend emotional therapy so that healing can be brought to your past in order to produce a better erection for tomorrow. Armed with the sum of this information, we will craft a plan together that will come up with a unique solution for your unique needs.

There is No One Size Fits All Solution

Just like there is no singular primary driver for erectile dysfunction, there is no one size fits all cure. As I mentioned before, it frustrates the physician in my soul to see doctors prescribe a pill after a 15-minute interview. You could build a city on the wasted months and years of men who thought there was no hope because the pill didn't work. A pill may very well be for you, but there is a good chance that it is a combination of treatments that will serve you best.

Injections could hold hope for the future of your erections, but it may take the addition of acoustic sound wave therapy to achieve the best result. It may be that a vacuum erectile device or a penis implant is necessary, but you do not want to travel that road unless you know all other options have been exhausted. Regardless of which path you choose, your diet and nutrition will always play a role. You can amplify the effects of any treatment with proper nutrition and supplementation.

If you have the "curved penis" disease, Peyronie's, then fret no longer. There is no reason that sexual experiences have to be full of fear, pain, or shame. You and your partner deserve the very best the human experience has to offer. Now you are one step away from a future without precedent. One step away, and it was the sum desire of this writing to encourage you to this next point.

Make an Appointment with Those Who Know

This is your next step, and it is remarkably simple. Armed with the information in this book, you need to make an appointment with someone who knows what they are talking about. I'm pleading with you, with all sincerity, to take this next step. For many of you, it may seem like you have been down this road before. You've made an appointment, only to cancel it out of embarrassment, and then finally show up and be prescribed a pill that never worked. Please, give it one more chance with someone who knows.

The rest of you have struggled with erectile dysfunction for some time now. Yet, for a variety of reasons, you have failed to take this next step. If that is the case for you, then do not worry. At least now, you know what to ask of your medical professional, and if they cannot speak this same language back to you, then stand up and walk straight out the door.

Now, I've been doing this for a long time, and I'd be remiss if I didn't suggest myself. If I can serve you in any way, please reach out to me immediately to schedule an office visit. However, if due to geography or other limiting factors, I cannot serve you in person, then please call me to schedule a phone consultation. If this is not possible, then find a local doctor who is on the same page. Find a doctor willing to go the distance with you, one that does a thorough intake. Find a doctor willing to talk to you about their own learning curve with treating erectile dysfunction. Sorry to say, but a doctor just doesn't walk out of medical school armed with the information you need to address this matter thoroughly.

Once again, I'm pleading with you, make yourself an appointment. That being said, you should be proud. You've just "made your bed" and accomplished the most important first task in this journey. You've done more than most men, and your partner thanks you for it. The Man Plan is designed for men who are ready to take that next step. The rest is up to you, and I hope to hear from each and every one of you soon. To a sexual future without precedent for you and for your partner. Let's get started.